Basics of Urinalysis

(Laboratory methods and techniques)

Ayman Mohamed

DEDICATION

I dedicate my book to my family and many friends. A special feeling of gratitude to my loving parents, Saber Mohamed and Karema Ramadan, whose words of encouragement and push for tenacity ring in my ears. I dedicate this work and give special thanks to my aunt Dr. Sohair R. Fahmi.

CONTENTS

ACKNOWLEDGMENTS

Firstly, I thank Allah for his grace, his success and his generosity. I take this opportunity to express my profound gratitude and deep regards to Dr. Sohair R. Fahmi, Associate Professor of Physiology, Zoology Department, Faculty of Science, Cairo University, for supervising the present work, his guidance, monitoring and constant encouragement during the work.
I would like to express my sincere gratitude to Dr. Amel Mahmoud Ali Soliman, Associate Professor of Physiology, Zoology Department, Faculty of Science, Cairo University, for her supervision, valuable advices, stimulating suggestions through this work.
Special thanks to Prof. Dr. Mohamed Assem Said Marie, Professor of Environmental Physiology, Zoology Department, Faculty of Science, Cairo University, for his help and support.
I deeply thank my family for their love, support and encouragement through the work.

CHAPTER 1: URINE COMPOSITIONS AND PHYSICAL EXAMINATION

Urinalysis

❖ Urinalysis is test that is done in order to analyze urine. Analysis of urine can provide important health clues.

❖ Urinalysis can be used to detect certain diseases, such as diabetes, gout, and other metabolic disorders, as well as kidney disease. It can also be used to uncover evidence of drug abuse.

❖ Consequently, urinalysis is an extremely valuable tool for demonstrating pathological conditions in the excretory system and as an index for the general metabolic condition of an individual.

Normal composition of urine

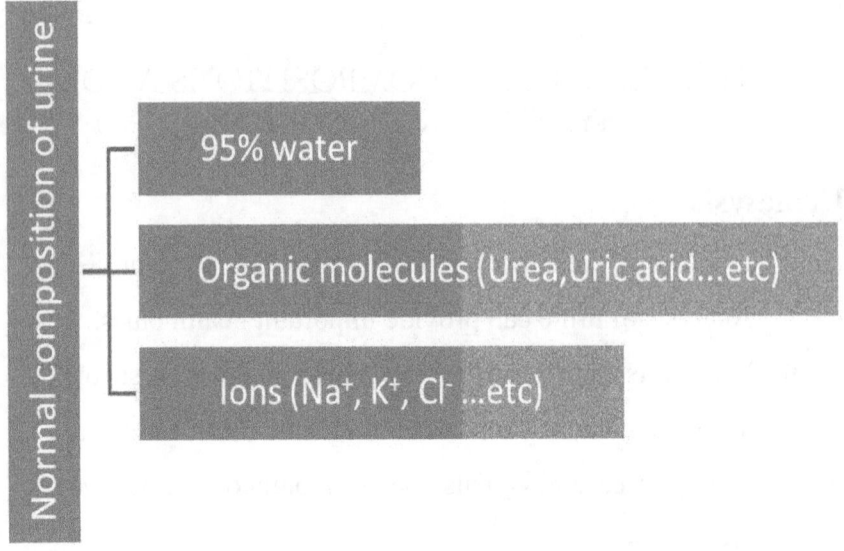

I. **Organic molecules**

1) **Urea**

❖ Urea is an organic compound whose chemical formula is $(NH_2)_2CO$.

❖ Urea is derived from ammonia and produced by the deamination of amino acids.

❖ The amount of urea in urine is related to quantity of dietary protein.

2) **Creatinine**

❖ Creatinine is produced mainly as a result of the breakdown of creatine phosphate in muscle tissue.

❖ It is usually produced by the body at a fairly constant rate (which depends on the muscle mass of the body).

3) Uric acid

❖ Uric acid is an organic compound whose chemical formula is: $C_5H_4N_4O_3$.

❖ It is produced mainly as a result of the breakdown of purines.

❖ Due to its insolubility, uric acid has a tendency to crystallize, and is a common part of kidney stones.

4) Other substances/molecules

❖ Example of other substances that may be found in small amounts in normal urine include carbohydrates, enzymes, fatty acids, hormones, pigments, and mucins (a group of large, heavily glycosylated proteins found in the body).

II. Ions

1) Sodium (Na^+)

❖ Amount in urine varies with diet and the amount of aldosterone (a steroid hormone) in the body.

2) Potassium (K^+)

❖ Amount in urine varies with diet and the amount of aldosterone (a steroid hormone) in the body.

3) Chloride (Cl^-)

❖ Amount in urine varies with dietary intake (chloride is a part of common salt, NaCl).

4) Magnesium (Mg^{2+})

❖ Amount in urine varies with diet and the amount of parathyroid hormone in the body. (Parathyroid hormone increases the reabsorption of magnesium by the body, which therefore decreases the quantity of magnesium in urine).

5) Calcium (Ca^{2+})

❖ Amount in urine varies with diet and the amount of parathyroid hormone in the body. (Parathyroid hormone increases the reabsorption of calcium by the body, which therefore decreases the quantity of calcium in urine.)

6) Ammonium (NH_4^+)

❖ The amount of ammonia produced by the kidneys may vary according to the pH of the blood and tissues in the body.

7) Sulphates (SO_4^{2-})

❖ Sulphates are derived from amino acids.

❖ The quantity of sulphates excreted in urine varies according to the quantity and type of protein in the person's diet.

8) Phosphates ($H_2PO_4^-$, HPO_4^{2-}, PO_4^{3-})

❖ Amount in urine varies with the amount of parathyroid hormone in the body - parathyroid hormone increases the quantity of phosphates in urine.

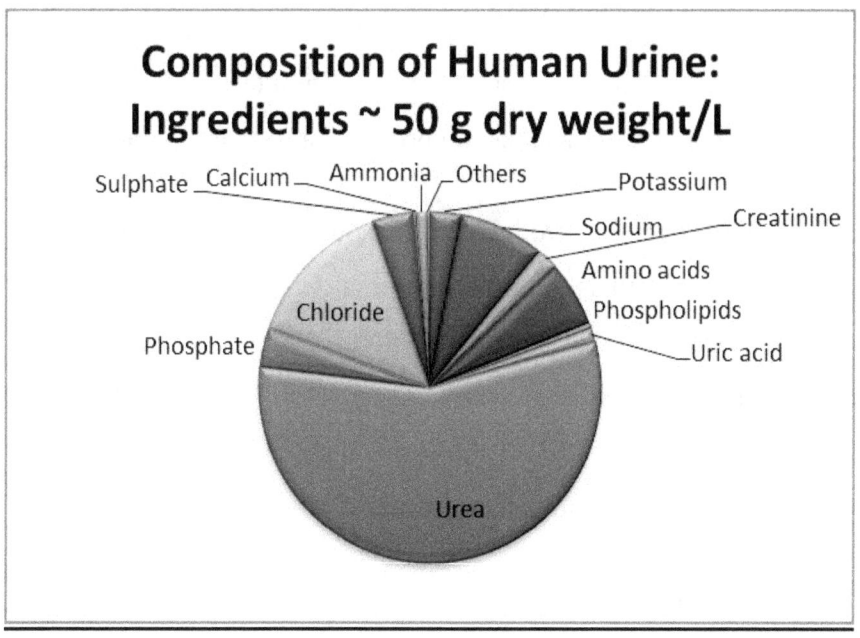

Abnormal composition of urine

1. Protein

❖ The protein test pad measures the amount of albumin in the urine.

❖ When urine protein is elevated, a person has a condition called proteinuria; this can be an early sign of kidney disease.

❖ Albumin is smaller than most other proteins and is typically the first protein that is seen in the urine when kidney dysfunction begins to develop.

❖ Other proteins are not detected by the test pad but may be measured with a separate urine protein test.

❖ Other conditions that can produce proteinuria include:

a) Disorders that produce high amounts of proteins in the blood, such as multiple myeloma
b) Conditions that destroy red blood cells
c) Inflammation, malignancies (cancer), or injury of the urinary tract - for example, the bladder, prostate, or urethra
d) Vaginal secretions that get into urine

2. Blood

❖ This test is used to detect hemoglobin in the urine (hemoglobinuria).

❖ Hemoglobin is an oxygen-transporting protein found inside red blood cells (RBCs). Its presence in the urine indicates blood in the urine (known as hematuria).

❖ The small number of RBCs normally present in urine usually result in a "negative" test. However, when the number of RBCs increases, they are detected as a "positive" test result.

❖ Even small increases in the amount of RBCs in urine can be significant.

❖ Numerous diseases of the kidney and urinary tract, as well as trauma, medications, smoking, or strenuous exercise can cause hematuria or hemoglobinuria.

❖ This test cannot determine the severity of disease nor be used to identify where the blood is coming from. For instance, contamination of urine with blood from hemorrhoids or vaginal bleeding cannot be distinguished from a bleed in the urinary tract. This is why it is important to collect a urine specimen correctly and for women to tell their health care provider that they are menstruating when asked to collect a urine specimen.

❖ Sometimes a chemical test for blood in the urine is negative, but the Microscopic Exam shows increased numbers of RBCs. When this happens, the laboratorian may test the sample for ascorbic acid (vitamin C), because vitamin C has been known to interfere with the accuracy of urine blood test results, causing them to be falsely low or falsely negative.

3. Glucose

❖ Glucose is normally not present in urine.

❖ When glucose is present, the condition is called glucosuria. It results from either:

a) Uncontrolled diabetes mellitus

b) A reduction in the "renal threshold." When blood glucose levels reach a certain concentration, the kidneys begin to excrete glucose into the urine to decrease blood concentrations.

c) Hormonal disorders, liver disease, medications, and pregnancy.

❖ High concentrations of ascorbate or ketoacids reduce test sensitivity. However, the degree of glycosuria occurring in diabetic ketoacidosis is sufficient to prevent false-negative results despite ketonuria.

4. Ketones

❖ Ketones are not normally found in the urine.
❖ They are intermediate products of fat metabolism.
❖ They can form when a person does not eat enough carbohydrates (for example, in cases of starvation or high-protein diets) or when a person's body cannot use carbohydrates properly.
❖ When carbohydrates are not available, the body metabolizes fat instead to get the energy it needs to keep functioning.
❖ Ketones in urine can give an early indication of insufficient insulin in a person who has diabetes.
❖ Severe exercise, exposure to cold, and loss of carbohydrates, such as with frequent vomiting, can also increase fat metabolism, resulting in ketonuria.
❖ False-positive results may occur in patients who are taking levodopa or drugs such as captopril or mesna that contain free-sulfhydryl groups.

5. Urobilinogen

❖ Urobilinogen is a colorless pigment normally present in urine in low concentrations.

❖ It is formed in the intestine from bilirubin, and a portion of it is absorbed back into the bloodstream.

❖ Positive test results help detect liver diseases such as hepatitis and cirrhosis and conditions associated with increased RBC destruction (hemolytic anemia).

❖ When urine urobilinogen is low or absent in a person with urine bilirubin and/or signs of liver dysfunction, it can indicate the presence of hepatic or biliary obstruction.

❖ Sulfonamides may produce false-positive results and degradation of urobilinogen to urobilin may yield false-negative results. Better tests are available to diagnose obstructive jaundice.

6. Bilirubin

❖ Bilirubin is not present in the urine of normal, healthy individuals.

❖ Bilirubin is a waste product that is produced by the liver from the hemoglobin of RBCs that are removed from circulation.

❖ It becomes a component of bile, a fluid that is secreted into the intestines to aid in food digestion.

❖ In certain liver diseases, such as biliary obstruction or hepatitis, bilirubin leaks back into the blood stream and is excreted in urine.

❖ The presence of bilirubin in urine is an early indicator of liver disease and can occur before clinical symptoms such as jaundice develop.

❖ False-negative results occur in the presence of ascorbate.

7. Nitrite

❖ This test detects nitrite and is based upon the fact that many bacteria can convert nitrate to nitrite in the urine.

❖ Normally the urinary tract and urine are free of bacteria.

❖ When bacteria find their way into the urinary tract, they can cause a urinary tract infection (UTI).

❖ Many bacteria can convert nitrate to nitrite in the urine.

❖ A positive nitrite test result can indicate a UTI. However, since not all bacteria are capable of converting nitrate to nitrite, someone can still have a UTI despite a negative nitrite test.

8. Leukocytes

❖ Leukocyte esterase is an enzyme present in most white blood cells (WBCs). Normally, a few white blood cells are present in urine and this test is negative.

❖ When the number of WBCs in urine increases significantly, this screening test will become positive.

❖ When the WBC count in urine is high, it means that there is inflammation in the urinary tract or kidneys.

❖ The most common cause for WBCs in urine (leukocyturia) is a bacterial urinary tract infection, such as a bladder or kidney infection.

❖ Contamination with vaginal debris may yield a positive test result without true urinary tract infection.

9. Indican

❖ Indican is an indole produced when bacteria in the intestine act on the amino acid, tryptophan.

❖ Most indoles are excreted in the feces.

❖ The remainder is absorbed, metabolized by the liver, and excreted as indican in the urine.

❖ Normally, only a small amount of indican is found in the urine.

❖ The amount of urine indican increases with high protein diets or inefficient protein digestion.

❖ If protein is not digested adequately, bacteria act on the protein causing putrefaction in the colon and the production of indoles, which are absorbed and converted in the liver to Indican.

❖ Conditions that lead to excess urine Indican include:

a) Maldigestion and/or malabsorption of protein

- Insufficient digestive enzymes (proteases such as trypsin, pepsin, chymotrypsin)

- Malabsorption syndromes (sprue, Hartnup disease, a rare disorder in which amino acids are poorly absorbed from the intestine, etc.)

b) Bacterial overgrowth in the small and/or large intestine

- intestinal obstruction
- concurrent intestinal parasitic infections
- concurrent intestinal fungal infection

c) Liver Dysfunction

❖ The inability to digest protein can have adverse effects on glycemic control, hormone balance and water balance.

Types of urine specimens

❖ Generally, about 10 mL of urine is required for routine urinalysis.

❖ Urine specimens should be refrigerated if they cannot be examined within 2 hours because urine begins to break down after that time, becoming more alkaline, and rendering some urine tests inaccurate.

1. **Random**

❖ A specimen obtained at any time during examination.

❖ This is the specimen most commonly sent to the laboratory for analysis, primarily because it is the easiest to obtain and is readily available.

❖ This specimen is usually submitted for urinalysis and microscopic analysis, although it can sometimes give an inaccurate view of a patient's health if the specimen is too diluted and analyte values are artificially lowered.

2. First morning specimen

❖ A specimen obtained during the first urination of the day.

❖ This is the specimen of choice for urinalysis and microscopic analysis, since the urine is generally more concentrated (due to the length of time the urine is allowed to remain in the bladder) and, therefore, contains relatively higher levels of cellular elements and analytes

3. Second-voided Specimen

❖ This is a specimen obtained after the first emptying of the bladder and waiting until a second voiding to collect the specimen.

❖ This is particularly useful for glucose as a specimen that has been maintained in the bladder for hours (such as overnight) may not accurately reflect glucose levels at the time the specimen is taken.

4. Two-hour postprandial

❖ This specimen is collected two hours after the patient has eaten a meal and requires only a clean container.

❖ The specimen is tested for glucose, and the results are used to monitor insulin therapy in patients with diabetes mellitus.

Special methods of urine collection

❖ When bacteriological studies are to be done, special collection techniques may be necessary to avoid contamination of the specimen.

1. Clean catch (Midstream)

❖ This is used for urine culture and cytological analyses.

❖ It may also be used for routine urinalysis in order to prevent contamination of the sample.

❖ It is obtained after cleansing about the urethral meatus with an antiseptic solution, such as benzalkonium hydrochloride.

❖ The first half of the urine flow is not collected in order to flush contaminants, but the collection cup captures the last half of the stream.

❖ Clean catch is especially important for females as it reduces contamination from vaginal secretions.

❖ Specimens obtained during menses should be clean catch and a tampon should be used, if possible, to prevent contamination of the specimen with menstrual fluids.

2. **Catheterized**

❖ Collection from Catheters **(e.g. Foley catheter)** using a syringe, followed by transfer to a specimen tube or cup. Alternatively, urine can be drawn directly from the catheter to an evacuated tube using an appropriate adaptor.

❖ This may be obtained with a straight catheterization or from an indwelling Foley catheter.

❖ If a Foley® catheter is in place, itis better to collect the sample directly from the catheter rather than the draining bag, but if protocol prevents disconnection, the drainage bag should be emptied and then a sample collected from fresh urinary drainage.

❖ Catheterization is avoided if possible because of the danger of trauma or introduction of infective agents. However, catheterization may be necessary for patients who are confused.

3. **Supra-pubic transabdominal needle aspiration**

❖ It may be necessary when a non-ambulatory patient cannot be catheterized or where there are concerns about obtaining a sterile specimen by conventional means.

❖ This method is used most commonly for infants or small children but may be used for bedridden patients who cannot be catheterized.

❖ It provides a very pure and sterile specimen.

4. Timed collection

❖ Among the most commonly performed tests requiring timed specimens are those measuring creatinine, urine urea nitrogen, glucose, sodium, potassium, or analytes such as catecholamines and 17-hydroxysteroids that are affected by diurnal variations.

❖ A timed specimen is collected to measure the concentration of these substances in urine over a specified length of time, usually 8 or 24 hours

❖ **Procedure for 24 hour collection:**

a) Begin collection in the morning, but do not save the first urination; however, record the time of urination as the beginning point.

b) Collect all urine is container provided by physician or laboratory (usually 4 L container with small amount of preservative).

c) Store the container in a refrigerator the entire 24 hours.

d) Urinate into small clean container and pour urine into the larger container.

e) Urinate at the end of the 24-hour period for the final time and save that specimen.

f) Record the final time.

g) Avoid getting any toilet paper, pubic hair, stool, menstrual blood, or other material in the urine.

h) Deliver to laboratory within 4 hours.

❖ In some cases, urine may be saved in two separate containers, one for daytime collection and the other for nighttime.

❖ For some conditions, longer specimen collection (up to 72 hours) may be indicated

5. Pediatric collection

❖ Pediatric Specimens present many challenges.

❖ For infants and small children, a special urine collection bag can be adhered to the skin surrounding the urethral area.

❖ The specimen is transferred to a sterile container immediately after the infant urinates.

Preservation of Urine Specimen

❖ Urine should be examined immediately as much as possible after it is passed, because some urinary components are unstable.

❖ If urine specimen cannot be examined immediately, it must be refrigerated or preserved by using different chemical preservatives.

❖ The maximum time that urinary content to be maintained in urine specimen is 2 hour.

❖ Long standing of urine at room temperature can cause:

- Growth of bacteia

- Break down of urea to ammonia by bacteria leading to an increase in the pH of the urine and this may cause the precipitation of calcium and phosphates.

- Oxidation of urobilingen to urobilin.

- Distruction of glucose by bacteria.

- Lysis of RBCs, WBCs and casts.

❖ **Method of Preservation of Urine Specimen**

1. **Refrigeration**

- The best general method of preservation up to 8 hours is refrigeration at 4-6°C. Refrigerated specimens are warmed to room temperature before performing an analysis.

2. **Toluene (Toluol)**

- If only the chemical contents of the urine are of interest, as with most 24-hour specimens, toluene may be used.

- Toluene merely lies on the surface of the urine, forming a thin layer and acting as a physical barrier to air and bacteria. However, anaerobic bacteria, if present, are not inhibited.
- To measure portions of the specimen, it is necessary either to remove the toluene or to pipet from below the surface.

3. Formalin (10 %)

- It is an excellent preservative for the formed (microscopic) elements in urine.
- About 4 drops of formalin may be used for each 100 ml of urine. However, it interferes with some qualitative chemical tests, and it should not be used when the glucose concentration is to be determined.

4. Boric Acid (0.8 %)

- Boric acid is a satisfactory preservative for general purposes.
- It will not interfere with examinations for protein, sugar, or ketone bodies.

5. Thymol (10 % in Isopropanol)

- Thymol is another general purpose preservative.
- Approximately 10 ml of the prepared solution is used for each 24-hour collection.

6. Chloroform

- Chloroform may be used as a preservative, but it interferes with some chemical tests and may cause cellular changes.

7. Sodium Fluoride

- Sodium fluoride may be used as a preservative for urine samples when one is concerned with glucose.
- It inhibits tests for glucose on the reagent strip.

8. Sodium Carbonate

- To preserve urobilinogen in urine requires special precautions.
- To assure alkalinity, a half-teaspoonful of sodium carbonate is placed in the specimen bottle before the urine is voided into the bottle.

Urine Specimen Handling Guidelines

1. Labels

- ❖ Include the patient name and identification on labels.
- ❖ Make sure that the information on the container label and the requisition match.

2. Volume

❖ Ensure that there is sufficient volume to fill the tubes and/or perform the tests. Underfilling or overfilling containers with preservatives may affect specimen-to-additive ratios.

3. Collection Date and Time

❖ Include collection time and date on the specimen label.

❖ This will confirm that the collection was done correctly.

❖ For timed specimens, verify start and stop times of collection.

❖ Document the time at which the specimen was received in the laboratory for verification of proper handling and transport after collection.

4. Collection Method

❖ The method of collection should be checked when the specimen is received in the laboratory to ensure the type of specimen submitted meets the needs of the test ordered.

❖ An example of an optimum specimen/test match would be a first morning specimen for urinalysis and microscopic examination.

5. Proper Preservation

❖ Check if there is a chemical preservative present or if the specimen has not been refrigerated for greater than two hours post collection.

❖ After accepting the test request, ensure that the method of preservation used is appropriate for the selected test.

❖ If the correct preservative was not used the test cannot be conducted.

6. **Light Protection**

❖ Verify that specimens submitted for testing of light-sensitive analytes are collected in containers that protect the specimen from light.

Type of Examination in Routine Urinalysis

❖ Urine analysis incudes three types of examination:

❖ Physical examination

❖ Chemical examination

❖ Microscopic examination

Type of Examination in Routine Urinalysis

Physical Examination	Chemical Examination	Microscopic Examination
Volume	Glucose	RBCs
Color	Protein	WBCs
Odor	Ketones	Epithelial cells
Appearance	Bilirubin	Casts
pH	Urobilinogen	Bacteria
Specific gravity	Blood	Yeasts
	Nitrite	Parasites
	Leukocyte Esterase	Crystals
	Indican	Artifacts

Physical Examination

1. **Color**

❖ Usually pale yellow/ amber and darkens

❖ Normal urine color varies from straw (light yellow color) to dark amber (dark yellow).

❖ Light yellow indicate that the urine is more diluted, and has low specific gravity. Such exceptional condition occurs in case of diabetic mellitus. In this condition the color of urine

23

is mostly light yellow, but because of having high glucose content, its specific gravity is high.

❖ On the other hand, dark amber (dark yellow) color mostly indicates that the urine is concentrated, and has high specific gravity.

❖ Normal urine color results from three pigments. They are:

    a) Urochrome, responsible for yellow color formation. This pigment is found in high proportion than the other two.

    b) Uroerythrin, responsible for red color formation.

    c) Urobilin, responsible for the orange-yellow color formation.

❖ Thus, normal urine gets its color from a combination of the above-mentioned three pigments.

❖ A variety of medications and other agents may cause the urine to change color.

❖ Patients taking medications that alter urine color should be advised to prevent alarm.

Color change	Clinical Implication
Pale to colorless	❖ Large fluid intake ❖ Diabetic mellitus ❖ Diabetic insipidus ❖ Alcohol consumption ❖ Nervousness
	❖ Concentrated urine ❖ Decreased fluid consumption ❖ Dehydration

Dark/brown	❖ Fever ❖ Certain urinary tract medication (eg. phenazophyridine) ❖ Yellow brown or "beer brown" color may indicate the presence of bilirubin.
Blue or blue green	Artificial food coloring Asparagus Hypercalcemia
Red/pink	❖ Blackberries ❖ Beets ❖ Blood (may relate to disease, exercise, or ❖ medications) ❖ Artificial food coloring ❖ Rhubarb ❖ Chronic lead or mercury ❖ poisoning

.

2. **Appearance**

❖ Should be clear but may be slightly cloudy.

❖ Cloudy urine (white or yellow) may be evidence of infection with pus or microscopic blood present, but it can also be caused by kidney stones, foods, vaginal discharge, and dehydration.

❖ Sometimes with urinary infections, long purulent strands may be noted in the urine specimen.

❖ **Clinical Implications**

a) White blood cells (pus cells) that occur due to UTI

b) Kidney stones

c) RBC's

d) Yeast cells,

e) High number of bacteria cells

f) High number of epithelial cells

g) Fat droplets in urine, which give opalescent appearance (rare condition).

h) Amorphous urates, in case of gout and leukemia.

i) High number of mucus trades.

❖ All the above findings are confirmed by urine microscopic examination.

3. **Odor**

❖ Normally fresh voided urine from healthy individuals has faint aromatic odor, which comes from volatile acids, normally found in urine, mostly, ammonia.

❖ Should be very slight, but some foods and medications, such as estrogen, may affect odor.

❖ Some bacteria may give urine a foul odor, depending upon the organism.

❖ Urine left at room temperature for more than 2 hours tends to develop an ammonia odor as bacteria converts urea into ammonia.

❖ If an ammonia odor is noted in a freshly voided specimen, this probably indicates that bacteria are active in the bladder, converting urea to ammonia.

❖ Some foods (such as asparagus), medications, and metabolic disorders may produce a strong or distinctive urine odor.

Odor	Clinical Significance
Sulfurous odor	Cystinuria and homocystinuria (type of amino acids, voided from abnormal metabolism)
Smell associated with the smell of a brewery (yeast)	Oasthouse urine disease
Cabbage like or "fishy" urine odor	Tyrosenemia
Aceton odor	Presence of ketone bodies in the urine, that may be due to diabetes mellitus, vomiting, starvation, strenuous exercise,

Sweat	Butyric / hexanoic acidemia produce a urine odor
Burnt sugar or maple	Maple sugar urine disease (infants, which has inherited amino acid metabolism disorder)

4. Volume

❖ Urine volume for a healthy adult is about 750 and 2500 mL of urine in 24 hours, or approximately 25 to 30 mL per hour.

❖ Children's output varies by age and size:

- Infants and toddlers: 2-3 mL/kg/hr.
- Preschool and young school age: 1-2 mL/kg/hr.
- School age and adolescents: 0.5-1 mL/kg/hr.

❖ Volume of urine excreted is related to:

a) Individual fluid intake

b) Body temperature

c) Climate

d) Individual's health status

Disorder	Definition	Clinical Significance
Polyuria.	Increased urinary output	❖ Diabetic mellitus ❖ Diabetic insipidus ❖ Certain tumors of brain and spinal cord Acromegaly
Oliguria	Excretion of constantly small amount of urine, i.e. below 400 ml of urine/24 hr	❖ Dehydration or poor blood supply to kidney that may be due to prolonged vomiting, diarrhea, etc. ❖ Obstruction of some area of the urinary tract/system (mechanical) ❖ Cardiac insufficiency ❖ Various renal diseases such as glomerulonephritis ❖ Fasting ❖ Excessive salt intake
Anuria	Complete absence of urine excretion or less than 100ml of urine per 24 hr.	❖ Complete urinary tract obstruction ❖ Acute renal failure ❖ Acute glomerulonephritis ❖ Hemolytic transfusion reaction

		❖ Polyuria may result physiologically after consumption of Intravenous glucose or saline Coffee, alcohol, tea, caffeine ❖ Pharmacological agent, such as thiazides and other diuretics

5. Specific Gravity

❖ Urinary specific gravity (SG) is a measure of the concentration of solutes in the urine.

❖ Specific gravity (SG), the ratio of the mass of a solution compared to the mass of an equal volume of water, is an estimate of the concentration of substances dissolved in the solution.

$$\text{Specific gravity} = \frac{\text{Weight of urine of measured volume}}{\text{Weight of distilled water of same volume}}$$

❖ The reference range is 1.005-1.030

❖ Low specific gravity (SG) (1.001-1.003) may indicate the presence of diabetes insipidus, a disease caused by impaired functioning of antidiuretic hormone (ADH).

❖ Low SG also may occur in patients with glomerulonephritis, pyelonephritis, and other renal abnormalities.

❖ In these cases the kidney has lost its ability to concentrate due to tubular damage.

❖ High SG may occur in patients with adrenal insufficiency, hepatic disease, congestive heart failure, or in patients experiencing excessive water loss due to sweating, fever, vomiting, or diarrhea.

6. **pH**

❖ Normal pH range: 5-6

❖ The kidneys strive to maintain the acid-base balance through reabsorption of sodium and tubular secretion of hydrogen and ammonium ions.

❖ The pH has an important role in the development of renal calculi.

❖ Acidic urine can result in xanthine, cystine uric acid, and calcium oxalate stones

❖ Alkaline urine can result in calcium carbonate, calcium phosphate, and magnesium phosphate stones.

Acidic urine	Alkaline urine pH
❖ High protein diet ❖ Acidosis ❖ Uncontrolled diabetes ❖ Diarrhea ❖ Starvation and dehydration ❖ Metabolic or respiratory acidosis	❖ Metabolic alkalosis (e.g., vomiting) ❖ Distal renal tubular acidosis ❖ Urea-splitting organisms (e.g., Proteus) (urine pH often ~9) ❖ Urine that is infected will become alkaline over time due to formation of ammonia (NH3) from bacterial urease ❖ Urine that is exposed to air for a long time can also have ❖ elevated pH due to loss of CO2 from the urine

Urine culture

❖ A urine culture is a test done in a laboratory to see whether urine has germs in it.

❖ A sample of midstream urine is put into a container.

❖ Then small plates with a growth medium that the germs can grow on are put into the sample and the container is closed tightly.

❖ The urine culture is then placed in an incubator for one to two days.

❖ If there are bacteria or fungi in the urine, visible colonies can grow.

❖ If bacteria are found during laboratory testing, then the type of antibiotic needed is usually determined at the same time.

Pregnancy tests

❖ Most tests can already determine whether a woman is pregnant eight to ten days after her period was due.

❖ They are usually done like rapid urine tests, using a urine sample in the morning after getting up.

❖ You can find exact instructions in the package insert.

❖ The urine of pregnant women contains a special hormone known as human chorionic gonadotropin (hCG), which is produced in the placenta.

❖ The results might be false if a woman does the test too soon, is taking medicine or drinks a lot of fluids before doing the test.

❖ Only a doctor can say for sure whether you are pregnant or not.

Other urine tests

❖ Drugs can also be detected in urine for a while after being used.

❖ Depending on the type of test, cannabis can be detected up to several weeks after being consumed.

❖ Drugs like cocaine, ecstasy or heroin can show up in test results for up to five days.

❖ Various types of tests can be used here too: Rapid tests help give police fast results on site, while other drug tests need to be sent to a laboratory.

❖ Urine samples can also be used to test athletes for banned performance-enhancing substances (doping).

CHAPTER 2: DETERMINATION OF CHEMICAL COMPOSITION OF URINE

I. Routine Dipstick Methodology

Principle

Proper tabs impregnated with chemical reagents are fixed to a plastic strip. Reagents are chromogenic altered with a chest, which is highly specific.

a. The procedure for using the dipstick is as follows:

b. Completely dip the test areas of the strip in fresh, well mixed, uncentrifuged urine and remove immediately.

c. Remove the excess urine from the stick by touching the edge of the strip to the urine container.

d. At the correct times, compare the test areas with the corresponding color charts on the container. The strip should be read in good lighting for accurate color comparison.

e. Record results as prescribed by your laboratory's protocol.

1. pH

❖ The pH test pads use indicator days that change color with pH.

❖ Physiologic urinary pH lies between 4.5 and 8.

❖ pH should be tested properly in freshly voided urine because:

- Growth of urea splitting bacteria and loss of carbondioxide (CO_2) raise the pH

- Bacterial metabolism of glucose may produce organic acids and lowers the pH

- These strips are not sufficiently accurate to be used for the diagnosis of renal tubular acidosis (RTA).

Principle:

❖ The test is based on the double indicator principle that gives a broad range of colors covering the entire urinary pH range.

❖ Colors range from orange through yellow and green to blue.

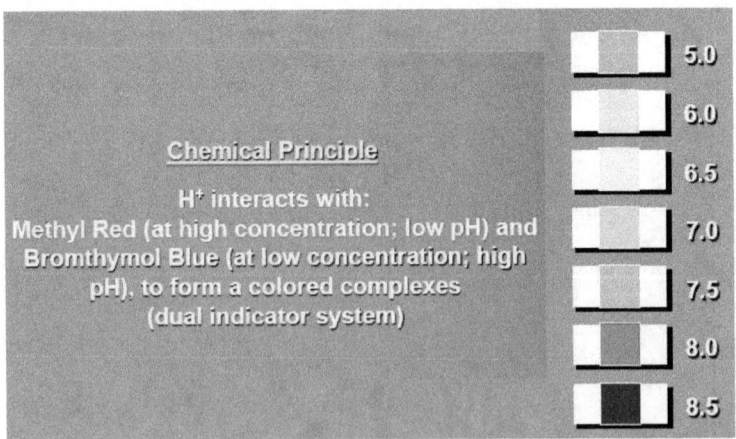

2. Protein

Principle:

❖ This test is based on the protein-error-of-indicators principle.

❖ At a constant pH, the development of any green color is due to the presence of protein.

❖ Colors range from yellow for "Negative" through yellow-green and green to green-blue for "Positive" reactions.

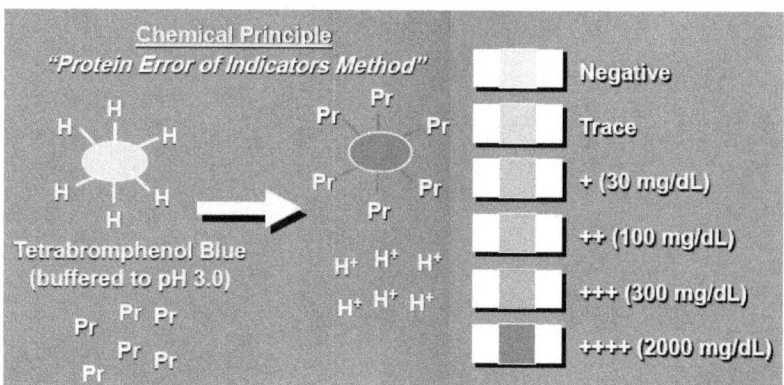

Microalbumin Dipstick

Albumin-selective dipsticks are available for screening for microalbuminuria in patients with incipient diabetic nephropathy. The most accurate screening occurs when first morning specimens are examined, because exercise can increase albumin excretion.

a) One type of dipstick uses colorimetric detection of albumin bound to gold-conjugated antibody.

❖ Normally, the urine albumin concentration is less than the 20 μg/L detection threshold for these strips.

❖ Unless the urine is very dilute, a patient with no detectable albumin by this method is unlikely to have microalbuminuria.

❖ Because urine concentration varies widely, however, this assay has the same limitations as any test that only measures concentration.

❖ This strip is useful only as a screening test and more formal testing is required if albuminuria is found.

b) A second type of dipstick has tabs for measurement of both albumin and creatinine concentration and permits calculation of the albumin-to-creatinine ratio.

3. Blood

Principle:

❖ This test is based on the peroxidase-iike activity of hemoglobin, which catalyzes the reaction of diisopropylbenzene dihydroperoxide and 3,3',5,5'-tetra methylbenzidine.

❖ The resulting color ranges from orange through green; very high levels of blood may cause the color development to continue to blue.

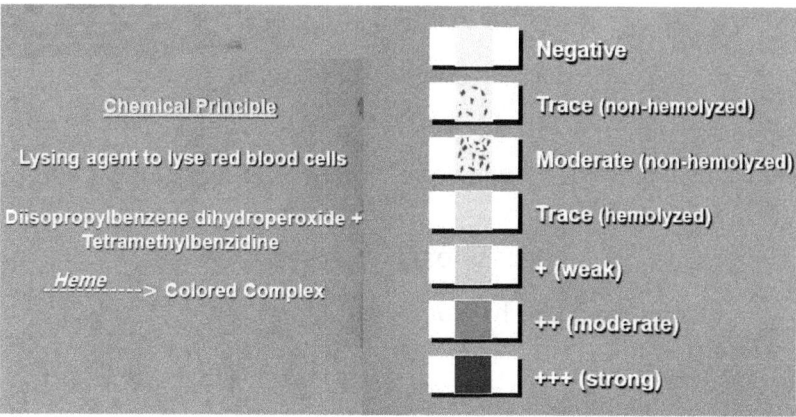

4. Specific Gravity

❖ This test is based on the apparent pKa change of certain pretreated polyelectrolytes in relation to ionic concentration.

❖ In the presence of an indicator, colors range from deep blue-green in urine of low ionic concentration through green and yellow-green in urines of increasing ionic concentrations.

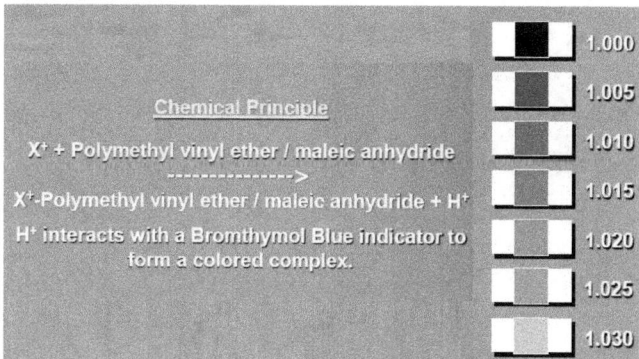

5. Glucose

Principle:

❖ This test is based on a double sequential enzyme reaction.

❖ One enzyme, glucose oxidase, catalyzes the formation of gluconic acid and hydrogen peroxide from the oxidation of glucose.

❖ A second enzyme, peroxidase, catalyzes the reaction of hydrogen peroxide with a potassium iodide chromogen to oxidize the chromogen to colors ranging from green to brown.

Chemical Principle		
		Negative
Glucose Oxidase		Trace (100 mg/dL)
Glucose + 2 H_2O + O_2 ---> Gluconic Acid + 2 H_2O_2		+ (250 mg/dL)
		++ (500 mg/dL)
Horseradish Peroxidase		+++ (1000 mg/dL)
3 H_2O_2 + KI ---> KIO_3 + 3 H_2O		++++ (2000+ mg/dL)

6. Ketones

Principle:

❖ This test is based on the development of colors ranging from buff-pink, for a negative reading, to purple when acetoacetic acid reacts with nitroprusside.

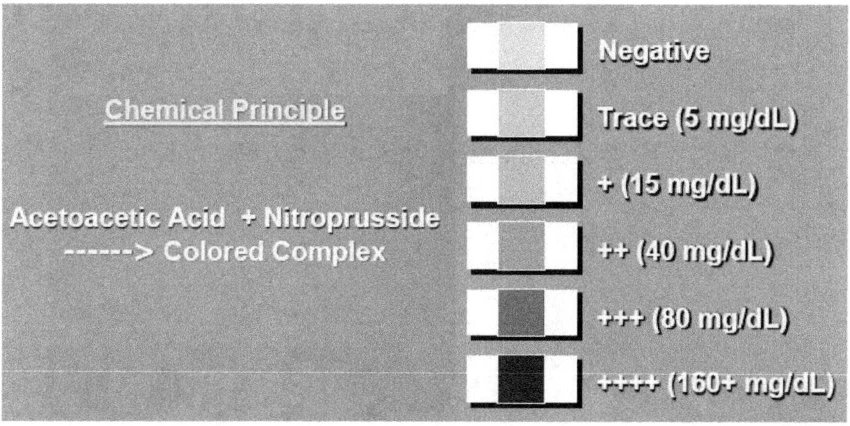

7. Urobilinogen

Principle:

❖ This test is based on a modified Ehrlich reaction, in which diethylaminobenzaldehyde in conjunction with a color enhancer reacts with urobilinogen in a strongly acid medium to produce a pink-red color.

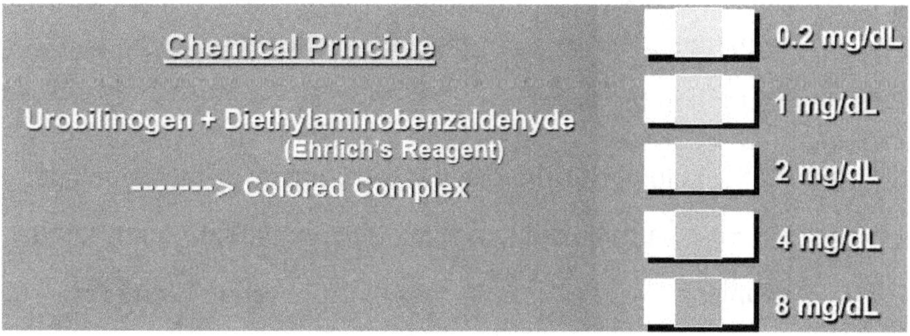

8. Bilirubin

Principle:

❖ This test is based on the coupling of bilirubin with diazotized dichloraniline in a strongly acid medium.

❖ The color ranges through various shades of tan.

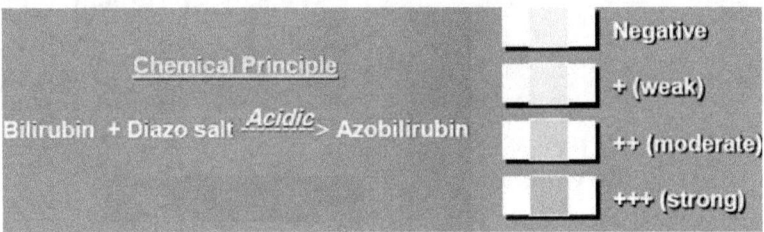

9. Nitrite

Principle:

❖ This test depends upon the conversion of nitrate (derived from the diet) to nitrite by the action of Gram negative bacteria in the urine.

❖ At the acid pH of the reagent area, nitrite in the urine reacts with p-arsanilic acid to form a diazonium compound in turn couples with 1,2,3,4-tetrahydrobenzoquinolin-3ol to produce a pink color.

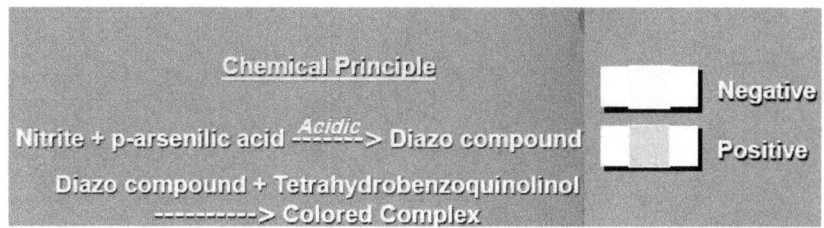

Chemical Principle

Nitrite + p-arsenilic acid $\xrightarrow{Acidic}$ Diazo compound

Diazo compound + Tetrahydrobenzoquinolinol
$\xrightarrow{\quad\quad}$ Colored Complex

Negative

Positive

10. Leukocytes

Principle:

❖ Granulocytic leukocytes contain esterases that catalyze the hydrolysis of the derivatized pyrrole amino acid ester to liberate 3-hydroxy-5-phenyl pyrrole.

❖ This pyrrole then reacts with a diazonium salt to produce a purple product.

❖ Non-granular WBC (lymphocytes) will not react with reagent strip reaction (false negative)

Chemical Principle		
Derivatized pyrrole amino acid ester		Negative
Esterases -----------> 3-hydroxy-5-phenyl pyrrole		Trace
		+ (weak)
3-hydroxy-5-phenyl pyrrole + diazo salt -------------> Colored Complex		++ (moderate)
		+++ (strong)

II. Chemical methods for urine examination

❖ The routine analysis of urine includes chemical test for protein, glucose, ketone bodies, occult blood, bile salts, bile pigments and urobilinogen .

A- Proteins in urine

All the methods are based on the principle of precipitation of protein by chemical agents or coagulation by heat.

Notes:

- If urine is alkaline make it slightly acidic by adding 3% glacial acetic acid.
- Turbid urine should be filtered or centrifuged and supernatant should be used

1- Heat and Acetic Acid Test

Procedures:

1. Place 5ml of clear urine in test tube
2. Boil the upper portion over a flame.
3. If turbidity develops add 1-2 drops of glacial acetic acid. Sometimes turbidity may be due to phosphate or carbonate precipitation. it is so then glacial acetic acid clear up the turbidity .if it is due to protein then precipitation will be there after the addition of acetic acid
4. Reboil the specimen
5. If turbidity is present protein is present, if there is no turbidity at upper portion then protein is absent.
6. Grade the turbidity as follows:

❖ Negative : No cloudiness
❖ Trace: Barely visible cloudiness.
❖ 1+ : definite cloud without granular flocculation
❖ 2+ : heavy and granular cloud without granular flocculation
❖ 3+ : dense cloud with marked flocculation.
❖ 4+ : thick curdy precipitation and coagulation

2- Sulphosalicyaclic Acid Test

Procedures:

1. Pipette 5 ml of urine into a clear test tube.
2. Add few drops of acetic acid
3. Add 5 drops of (30%) sulfosalicylic acid solution to the urine.

4. Compare with a tube of untreated urine against a black background.

5. Turbidity is graded as follows:

- ❖ Trace cloudiness against dark background
- ❖ 1+: dense cloudiness.
- ❖ 2+: cloudiness with granules and definite flocculation.
- ❖ 3+: cloudiness with flocculation.
- ❖ 4+: cloudiness with precipitation.

3- Nitric acid test

1. Add 3 ml of HNO_3 in test tube
2. Add urine on the wall of test tube
3. White ring appears at the junction of two liquids

B- Sugar in Urine

1- Benedicts Test

Principle:

- ❖ When benedicts qualitative reagent is heated with 8 drops of urine glucose present in urine reduces cupric ions present in reagent to cuprous ions.
- ❖ Alkaline medium is provided to the reaction by sodium carbonate present in reagent the color changes to green yellow orange or red according to concentration of glucose in urine.

Benedict's reagent:

- ❖ Sodium citrate   1.73 gm.
- ❖ Sodium bicarbonate 100 gm.
- ❖ Place in about 900 ml of distilled water.
- • Boil for 2-3 minutes and add 17.3 gm of cupric sulfate
- • Make final volume up to 1 liter
- • The reagent is stable at room temperature.

Procedure

1. Pipette 3 ml of benedicts reagent in test tube
2. By using Pasteur pipette add 5ml of urine
3. Heat carefully or place in boiling water bath for 5mins
4. The color is graded as follows:

- ❖ No change in color i.e. blue: Absence of sugar.
- ❖ Pale green with slightly cloudy: Trace
- ❖ Definite cloudy green: 1+
- ❖ Yellow to orange precipitate with supernatant fluid pale blue: 2+
- ❖ Orange to red precipitate supernatant fluid pale blue: 3+
- ❖ Brick red precipitate supernatant decolorized: 4+

2- Fehling's reaction

Procedures:

1- Add to the tube 1 ml of urine, and an equal volume of Fehling solution.

2- The content of the tube is heated.

3- In the beginning the color of the solution is yellow, and more heated it becomes red.

3- Nilender's reaction

Procedures:

1- Add into the test tube 1 ml of pathological urine, 1 ml of Nilender's reagent (which contains bismuth salt), and place the tube in a boiling water bath.

2- After a few minutes, the liquid begins to get darker glucose reduces $Bi(OH)_3$ until free bismuth and black precipitate are formed.

3- This reaction is sensitive and allows detecting glucose even when its concentration is low (about 0.5 g/l).

4- Fischer reaction

❖ Glucose, lactose, and other carbohydrates with a free aldehyde group (reducing carbohydrates), heated with an excess of phenyl hydrazine, form ozazones, nearly insoluble crystals of various shape.

❖ During the reaction of phenyl hydrazine with glucose, crystals in the shape of a whisk, and with lactose in the shape of sea urchins are formed.

❖ Usually, this reaction is used to distinguish between glucose and lactose. However, it can be used to identify other monosaccharides on the basis of the different melting temperatures of their ozazones: glucozazons, fructozazons melt at +210 °C, galactozazon melts at +180 °C, and pentozazons melt at +160 °C.

Procedure:

1. Add into the tube 0.3 g of phenyl hydrazine, 0.1 g of sodium acetate (CH₃COONa), a drop of glacial acetic acid and 1 ml of urine.

2. Place the tube for 30 minutes in a boiling water bath and then rapidly cool its content to fall out yellow crystals of ozazones (the crystals are examined under a microscope).

5- The Selivanov reaction

❖ It is used to detection of fructose.

❖ During the reaction of fructose with hydrochloric acid, oxymethyfurfural is forming, which reacts with resorcinol to form a red colored compound.

❖ With aldoses this reaction is very slow.

Procedure

1. Add into the tube 1 2 ml of the Selivanov reagent (0.05 g resorcinol in 100 ml of 20% hydrochloric acid) and 1 ml of urine.

2. The tube is placed in a boiling water bath.

3. The boiling content of the tube turns red.

C- Ketone bodies

1- Legal's reaction

❖ The reaction of acetone and acetoacetic acid with sodium nitroprusside in an alkaline medium gives a red orange coloured complex compound.

❖ The addition of acetic acid changes the structure of the complex, and its red-orange colour turns cherry.

Procedures:

1- Add to the test tube containing 3 ml of urine 5 drops of 10% $Na_2Fe(CN)_5NO$ and 1 ml of 10% NaOH; they give an orange color

2- Adding 2 ml of concentrated acetic acid, color turns cherry.

2- Rothera's test

❖ Nitroprusside used in this test reacts with both acetone and acetoacetic acid in presence of alkali (NH_4OH) to produce permanganent calomel red ring at the junction

Procedures:

1. Transfer about 5 ml of urine to a test tube
2. Saturate with ammonium sulphate
3. Few drops of 20% sodium nitroprusside
4. Layer the liquor NH_4OH on the side of the tube
5. Observe permanganate calomel ring at the junction of two layers.

3- Chemical test for detection aceto-acetic acid

Procedures:

1- Add dil.solution of $FeCl_3$ in test tube

2- Add 5 ml of urine

3- Deep red color is obtain

D- Bile in Urine

Bilirubin, bile salt, bile pigment, urobilin, urobilinogen are the constituents of bile.

1. Hay's test (Determination of Bile Salt)

Principle:

- ❖ Bile salts when present lower the surface tension of urine and sulphur powder is added to the urine, sulphur particles sink to the bottom of the tube.
- ❖ In the case of normal urine, it will float on the surface.

Procedures:

1. Place about 10 ml of urine in a test tube
2. Sprinkle a little dry sulphur powder on to the surface of urine.
3. Observe sulphur particles.

2. Fouchet's test for bile pigments

Principle

❖ When barium chloride is added to urine it combines with sulphate radicals in urine and precipitate of barium phosphate is formed.

❖ If bile pigments are present in urine, they will adhere to these large molecules.

❖ Ferric chloride present in Fouchet's reagent then oxidizes yellow bilirubin in presence of trichloroacetic acid to green bilverdin.

Fouchet's reagent:

❖ Trichloroacetic acid   25 gm

❖ Distilled water   100 ml

❖ % 10ferric chloride solution   10 ml

Procedures:

1. Add 10 ml of urine to 2.5 ml of barium chloride in test tube
2. Filter
3. Unfold the filter paper and spread it on the dry filter paper.
4. Allow 1 drop of Fauchet's reagent on the precipitate
5. A green or blue color indicates presence of bilirubin.

3. Ehrlichs aldehyde test for urobilinogen

Ehrlich's reagents:

❖ Paradimethylaminobenzaldehyde   2 gms.

❖ %20HCl   100 ml.

Procedures:

1. Take 5 ml of urine in test tube and add half volume about 2.5 ml of barium chloride.

2. Mix well and filter.

3. Take 2.3 ml of filtrate and add 0.5 ml of aldehyde reagent.

4. Allow to stand for 3 mins.

5. View the top column of urine against a white background.

6. A pink color denotes the presence of urobilinogen.

4. Schlesingers Test for Urobilin

Procedures:

1. Take 10 ml of urine and 6 drops of tincture of iodine in test tube (A).

2. Take 1 gm of powdered zinc acetate and 10 ml 95% alcohol in another test tube (B)

3. Mix by pouring A intoB and vice versa repeatedly until the solid zinc acetate has mostly gone into solution.

4. A green color is due to compound of zinc with urobilin

E- Blood

❖ Blood may be present in the urine as either red blood cells or hemoglobin.

❖ If enough blood is present the color of sample may be range from pink tinged to red to brownish black.

1. **Benzidine Test**

Principle:

❖ The peroxidase activity of hemoglobin present in urine decomposes hydrogen peroxide and the liberated oxygen oxidized benzidine to form a green- blue colored complex.

Procedures:

1. Dissolve some benzidine crystals in 0.5 ml of glacial acetic acid

2. Add 1 ml of urine, and a few drops of H_2O_2 and observe the color.

F- Indican

Procedures:

1. Add 5ml of urine to equal volume of mixture of (0.2% $FeCl_3$ and Conc.HCl)

2. Add 2ml of chroloform and shake vigorously.

3. Purple color is developed in chroroform layer.

CHAPTER 3: MICROSCOPIC EXAMINATION OF URINE

❖ As part of a urinalysis, the urine sediment is centrifuged and examined microscopically for crystals, casts, red blood cells, white bloods cells, and bacteria or yeast.

❖ Because examination of urinary sediment provides a direct sampling of urinary tract morphology, it provides important information useful for both diagnosis and prognosis.

❖ Microscopic examination of urine sediment is usually performed in addition to routine procedures.

❖ This examination requires a degree of skill acquired through practice under the immediate supervision of an experienced technician.

❖ The specimen used for microscopic examination should be as fresh as possible.

I. RED BLOOD CELLS

❖ **Normal:** 0-3 RBC/hpf (identified on high power due to their small size)

❖ Abnormal RBC: damage to basement membrane of glomerulus, kidney infection, kidney stones, trauma

❖ RBC in urine called hematuria

❖ Identification:

a. Smooth biconcave discs (~ 7 microns), no nucleus

b. Cells crenate in hypertonic (concentrated) urine

c. Cells swell and lyse in hypotonic (dilute), alkaline urine

❖ Other substances confusing with RBCs:

1. **Yeast**

   Tend to be spherical or ovoid, vary in size, often show 'budding'; add 2% acetic acid to differentiate (RBC hemolyze, yeast will not hemolyze)

2. **Oil droplets or air bubbles**

   Variations in size (RBC uniform in appearance)

3. **Oval form of calcium oxalate crystal**

   Add 2% acetic acid, RBC will hemolyze

4. **WBC in hypertonic (concentrated) urine**

   WBC loses water, become smaller; add 2% acetic acid to enhance nucleus (in hypertonic urine, crenated RBC)

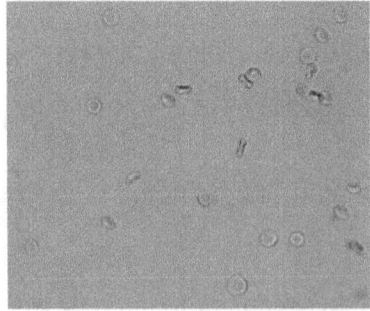 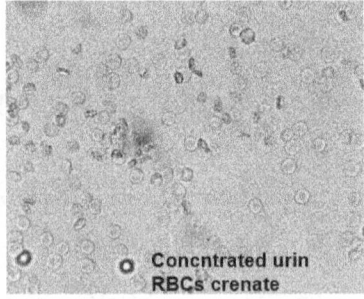

Concentrated urin RBCs crenate

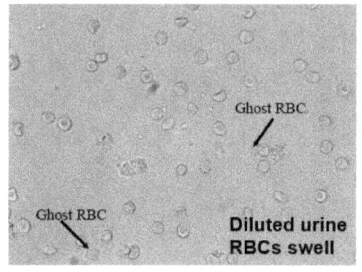

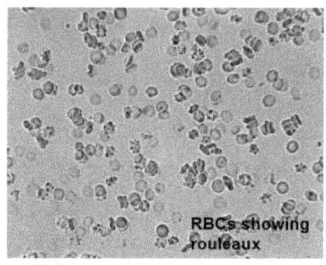

II. Leukocytes (WBCs)

❖ **Normal range**: 0-4 WBC/HPF.

❖ Since neutrophils are the predominant WBC in plasma, neutrophils are the predominant cell in urine

❖ **Identification of Neutrophils**:

a. Spherical , granules in cytoplasm, lobed (segmented) nucleus

b. ~10-14 microns in diameter (roughly 2x larger than RBC)

c. Can be found singly or aggregated in clumps (hard to enumerate)

d. Hypotonic (dilute) urine:

- Swell and become spherical balls that lyse rapidly

- Glitter cells: swollen WBCs showing Brownian movement

e. Hypertonic (concentrated) urine: become smaller, but do not crenate (use 2% acetic acid to differentiate from crenated RBCs)

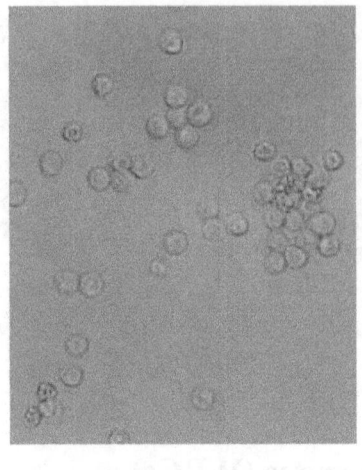 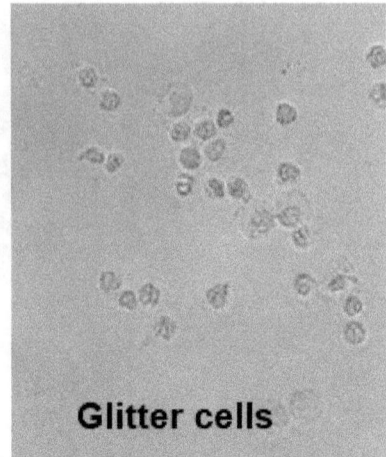

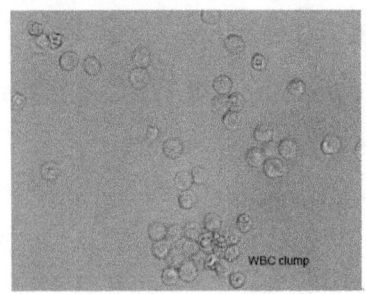 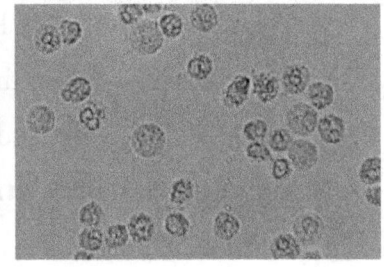

III. Epithelial cells

❖ **Normally** few epithelial cells (0-2 / HPF) can be found

❖ **Appearance:** their size differs depending on the site from which they originated.

❖ **Significance:** Epithelial cells are seen in urine due to sloughing of old cells from the lining of the genitourinary system or from damage caused by inflammatory process or renal disease

1. **Squamous cells**

   ❖ Originate in the superficial lining of the urethra and vagina

   ❖ Most common type of epithelial cell found in urine.

   ❖ Increased numbers may be seen as a contaminant in females indicating improper collection technique.

   ❖ This type of epithelial cell is 'not exclusively renal', and usually is diagnostically insignificant.

   ❖ Largest epithelial cell (40-60 microns) and thus identified on low power

   ❖ Clue Cells:

   ▪ Squamous epithelial cells with large amount of bacteria adhering to them giving them a shaggy' appearance

   ▪ Originates in vaginal mucosa, so considered vaginal contaminant; presence indicates bacterial vaginal infection

   ❖ Shape:

   a. Thin and flat having a 'flagstone' appearance, with distinct edges.

   b. Small centrally located nucleus with small amount of cytoplasm (fried egg appearance); can be a-nucleated

   c. Fine granulation in cytoplasm which becomes more dense with degeneration

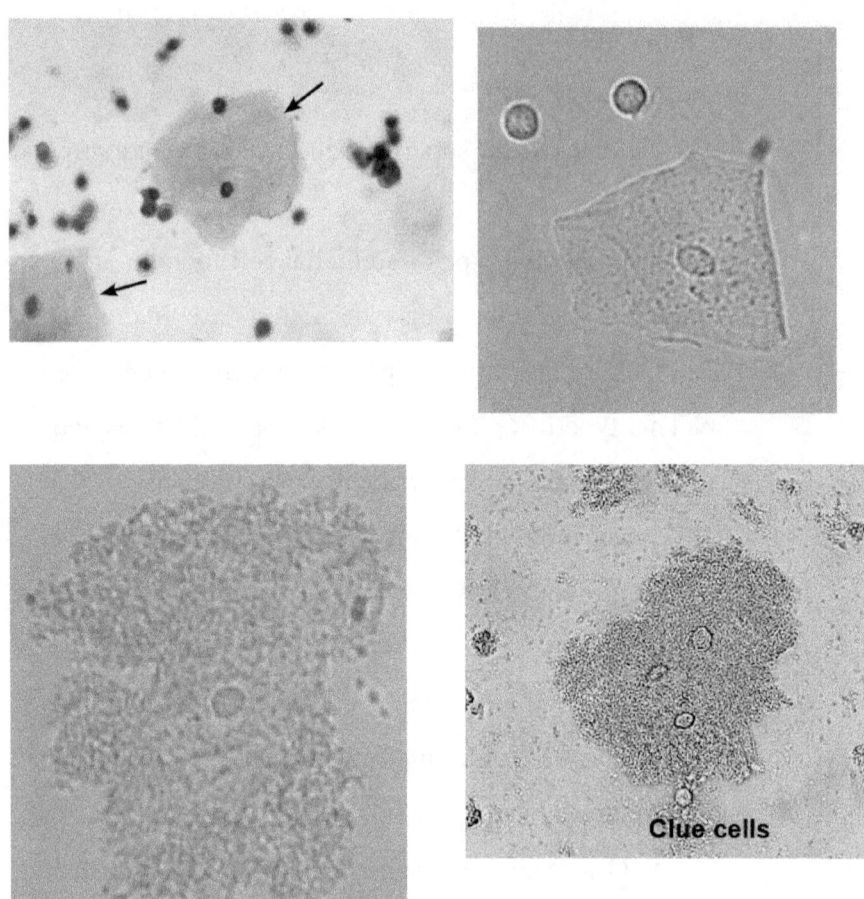

Clue cells

Clue cells

2. Transitional (urothelial) cells

❖ Originate in the lining of the renal pelvis, ureters, bladder and upper urethra.

❖ Normal to see few in urine as a result of normal sloughing.

❖ Seldom pathologically important unless large numbers exhibiting unusual morphology is seen

❖ Vary in size depending upon their location in urinary tract; evaluated using high power

❖ 30-40 micron in size (a little bit larger than a WBC)

❖ Evaluate and enumerate using high power objective

❖ Shape:

a. Round or pear-shaped; dense oval-to-round nucleus about the same size of a RBC or WBC.

b. Abundant cytoplasm : nucleus to cytoplasm ratio is approximately 1:5

c. The peripheral borders of the nucleus and cytoplasm are distinctly outlined.

d. Cells originating from intermediate layers of epithelium appear smaller, rounder (20-30 micron)

e. Cells originating from the single basal layer of epithelium tend to be elongated or columnar

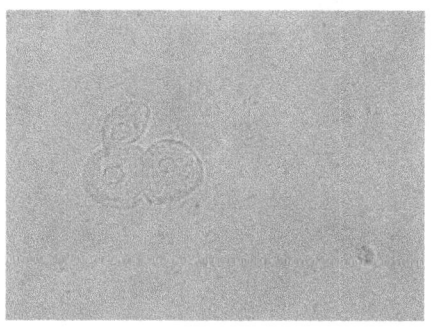 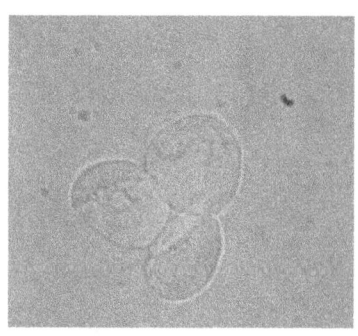

3. Renal tubular cells

❖ Originate in the linings of the renal tubules.

❖ Renal tubular cells are the most significant as increased numbers indicate tubular necrosis (pathology).

❖ Normal to see few in urine as a result of normal sloughing.

❖ Newborn infants have more renal tubular cells in urine as compared to older children and adults

❖ Vary in shape depending upon location in urinary tract; only epithelial cell that is renal in origin; evaluated using high power

❖ Shape:

    a. Round and slightly larger than WBC

    b. Nucleus with dense chromatin pattern, usually eccentric; can be multinucleated

    c. Nucleus to cytoplasm ratio approx. 1:1

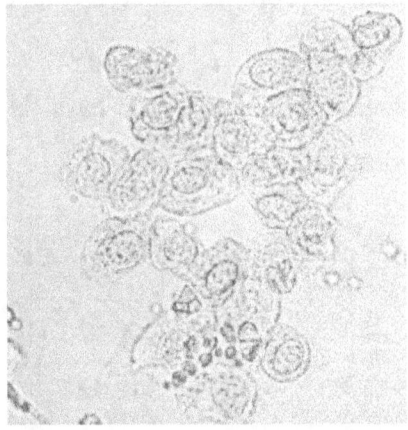

Oval Fat Bodies (OFB)

❖ Renal tubular epithelial cell with absorbed fat

❖ Highly refractive due to absorbed fat; amount of absorbed fat varies

❖ May also see free floating fat droplets

❖ Indicates pathology: evaluate and enumerate using high power objective

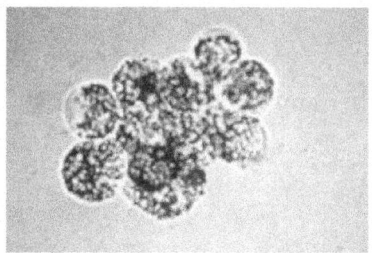 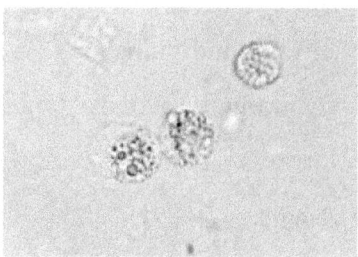

IV. Casts

❖ These urinary sediments are formed by coagulation of albuminous material in the kidney tubules.

❖ Casts are only formed in the kidney tubules: not the bladder, not urethra, not ureters

❖ If casts are present in large numbers, the urine is almost sure to be positive for albumin.

❖ Enumerated using low power and identified/classified using high power

❖ Significance:

Casts reflect status of renal tubules; extent and severity of renal disease correlates with type and number of casts present.

❖ Increased numbers usually seen with increased urinary protein levels (due to a glomerular problem) or urinary stasis (due to a blockage or disease)

❖ Normal: few hyaline or granular casts can be seen in normal individuals

❖ Abnormal: increased number and type; certain casts are always pathologic

❖ Shape:

    a. Since casts are formed in the tubules, casts are cylindrical with parallel sides and vary in length and width (cigar, submarine shape)

    b. Ends may be round, blunt or broken

    c. May have cellular components included inside the cast

    d. Wider if formed in collecting ducts: called broad casts

    e. Casts can be confused with mucus threads, fibers

❖ The 'youngest' cast is the hyaline and the 'oldest' cast is the waxy cast

❖ Structural Makeup of Casts

    ▪ Consists of a uromodulin matrix

    ▪ Uromodulin is a glycoprotein formerly called the Tamm-Horsfall protein

    ▪ This protein matrix does not react with the protein reagent strip test

❖ There are seven types of casts. They are as follows:

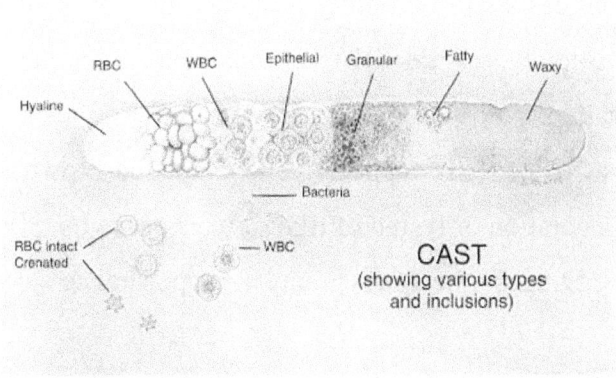

CAST
(showing various types
and inclusions)

1. Hyaline Casts

❖ Homogenous matrix, acellular (or may have few granules)

❖ Cylindroid = hyaline with a tail at one end, not significant

❖ Can be confused with mucus thread

❖ Most commonly observed cast: normally 0-2 / lpf

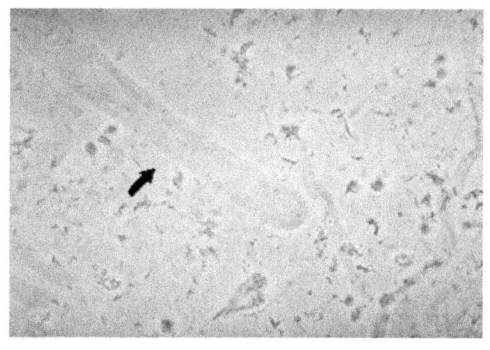
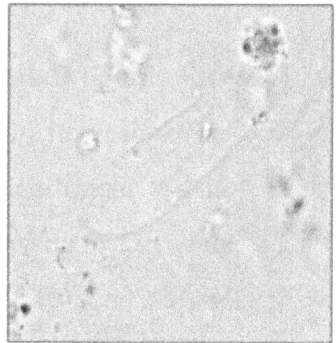

2. Red Blood Cell Casts

❖ Contain clearly discernible RBC's.

❖ Some casts will be tightly packed with RBC's, others may have only several RBC's contained in protein matrix (hyaline)

❖ Cast color may appear yellow to red-brown (due to degeneration or lysing of RBC as cast ages)

❖ As cast ages it becomes granular in appearance

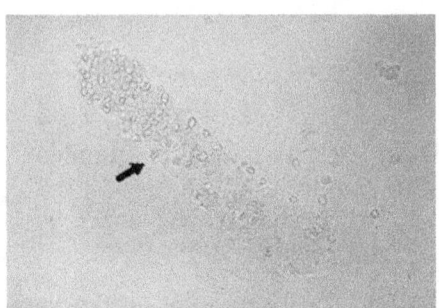 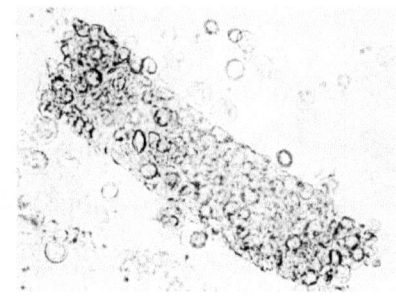

3. White Blood Cell Casts

❖ Consist of white blood cells in the protein matrix (hyaline)

❖ Readily identifiable, unless WBC are degenerating; then can be misidentified as renal tubular epithelial cell cast.

❖ The presence of WBC, free-floating or in clumps, in the urine can suggest strongly that the cast is a WBC cast.

❖ Lobed nucleus for WBC cast, and nucleus to cytoplasm ratio 1:1

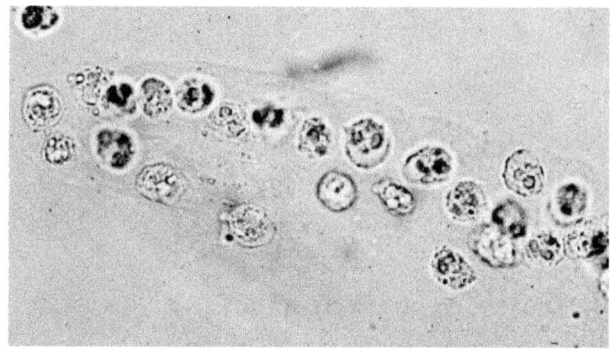

4. Epithelial Cell Casts

❖ Consist of renal tubular cells (RTE) in the protein matrix (never squamous or transitional)

❖ Can be misidentified as WBC cast; staining and phase microscopy needed to look at the nucleus to distinguish if RTE or WBC cast

❖ Look for nucleus to cytoplasm ratio 1:1 for RTE cast, lobed nucleus for WBC cast

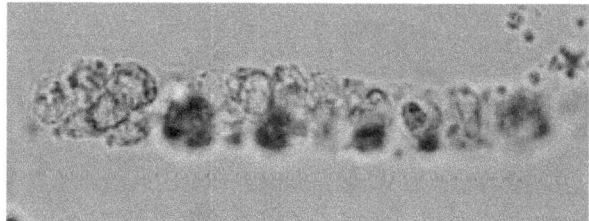

5. Granular Casts

❖ May appear as finely or coarsely granular, no intact cells are visible.

❖ Seen in renal disease; cause of granular cast formation varies: pathologic

❖ Cellular cast that has remained in tubule due to urine stasis (cells degenerate to granules)

❖ Degeneration of RTE cells that have released intracellular components that become enmeshed into cast matrix

❖ Can see occasional fine granular cast in normal individuals, following exercise or stress.

❖ These granular casts are unrelated to cellular casts

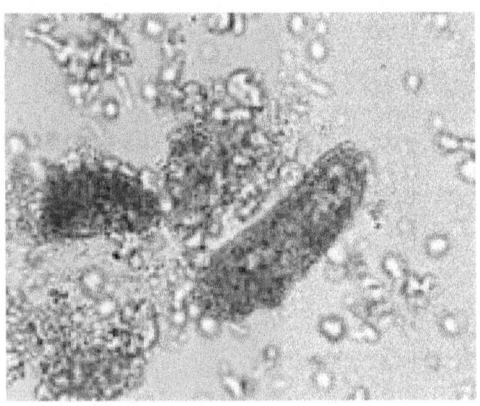

6. Waxy Casts

❖ Highly refractive, with a homogenous texture, well defined edges, and blunt, uneven ends

❖ Often see cracks along the length of the cast

❖ Appear yellow, grayish or colorless

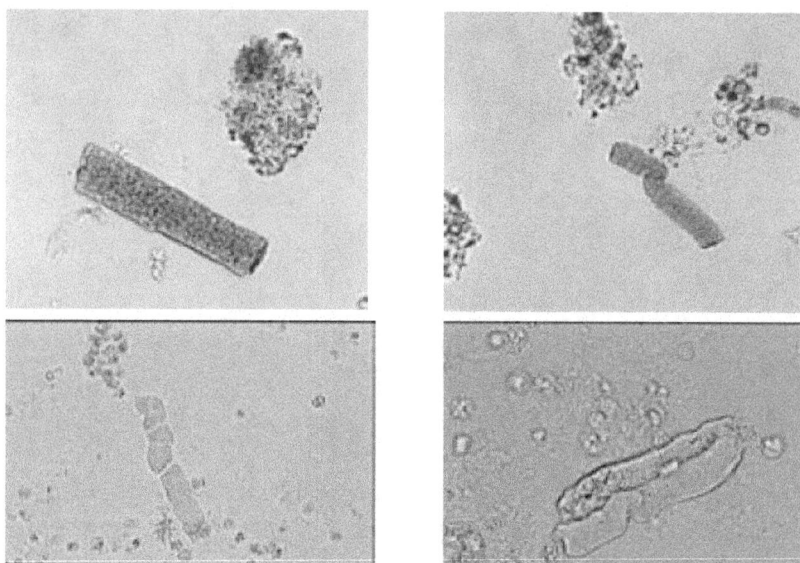

7. Fatty Casts

❖ Highly refractive due to fat content

❖ Contain free fat globules inside cast matrix (hyaline, granular)

❖ Fat globules appear light yellow to brown

❖ Can use Sudan III or Oil Red O stain (triglycerides stain orange-red; cholesterol does not) (textbook, figure 8-4)

❖ Found in numerous renal diseases, especially nephrotic syndrome and significant proteinuria; severe crushing injury with disruption of body fat. Pathologic

Ayman Mohamed

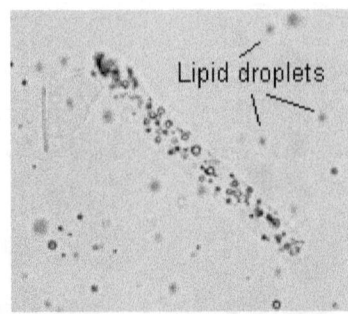

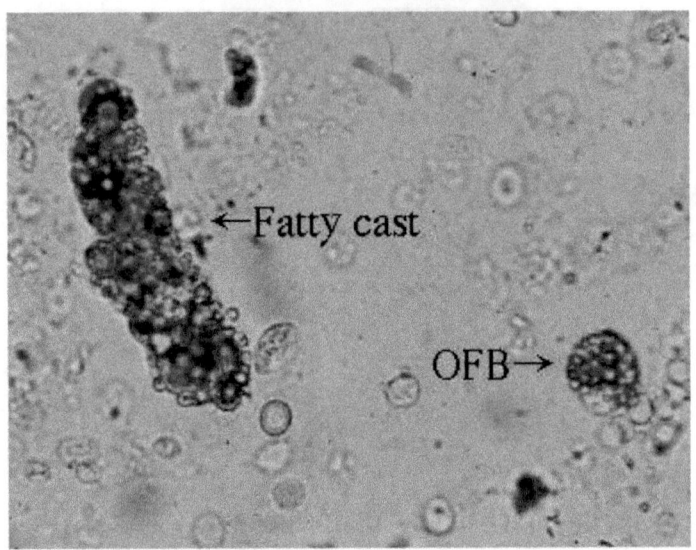

V. <u>Crystals</u>

❖ Not normally found in fresh urine

❖ If found in fresh urine, pathologic

❖ Crystals precipitate as urine cools to room temp or when urine is refrigerated

❖ All clinically significant crystals are found in acid urine

❖ Crystal Formation Enhanced By

- Increased concentration of solute in urine

- Urine pH
- Urine stasis
- Temperature

Normal crystals found in acid urine

1. Amorphous urates

❖ Urate salts (sodium, potassium, magnesium, calcium) can precipitate in amorphous (non-crystalline) forms

❖ Microscopically appear as small yellow-brown 'sand-like' granules

❖ Uroerythrin (pigment) readily deposit on these granules giving sediment a pink-orange or 'brick-dust' color

❖ Formation enhanced with refrigeration of urine

❖ Readily dissolve at alkaline pH or heating to 60°C; will form uric acid crystals when concentrated acetic acid added

❖ Very similar to amorphous phosphates: use pH to differentiate

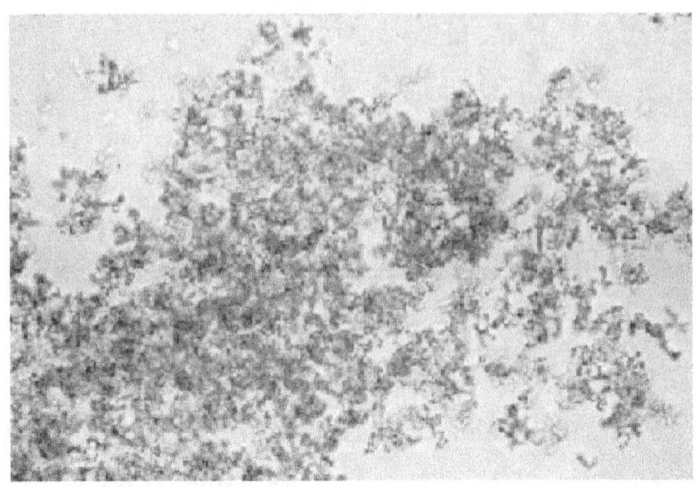

2. Uric acid

❖ Occur in several forms (pleomorphic), singly or clusters and layer or laminate on top of one another

❖ Yellow to orange-brown color with intensity depending on thickness of crystal; multicolored when polarized.

❖ Diamond shape most common form; rhombic plates, rosettes, wedges, needles, barrels; can be misidentified as cystine crystals when they have six sides

❖ Usually considered a 'normal crystal' but can be associated with gout and chemotherapy

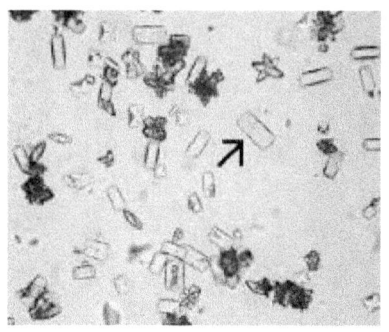
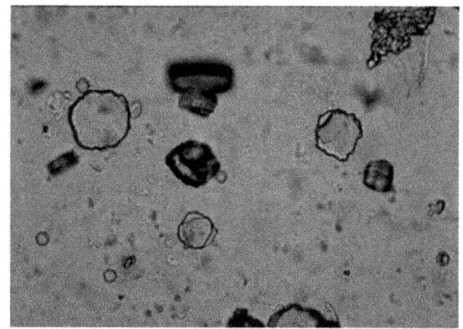
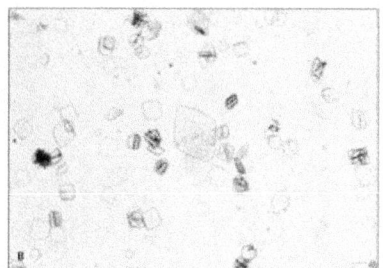
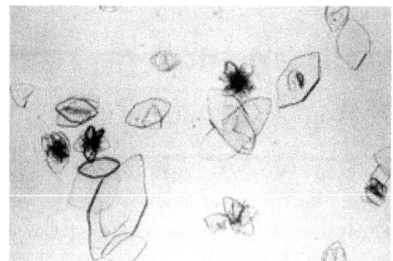

3. Calcium oxalate

❖ Most frequently observed crystal in urine; most common form is octahedral or envelope shape; size varies

❖ Small, ovoid or dumbbell shape is less common; can be misidentified as RBC (add 2% acetic acid to differentiate, RBC will hemolyze)

❖ Multicolored when polarized

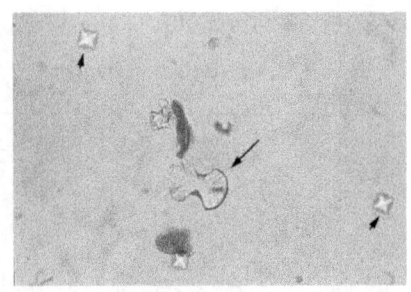 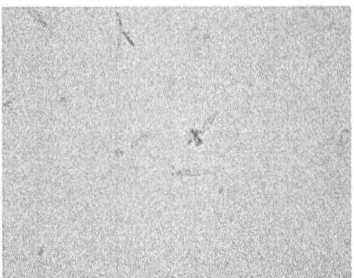

4. Hippuricacid

❖ Acid and neutral pH

❖ Rarely seen in urine

❖ Little to no clinical significance

❖ Clear to yellow-brown prisms /plates

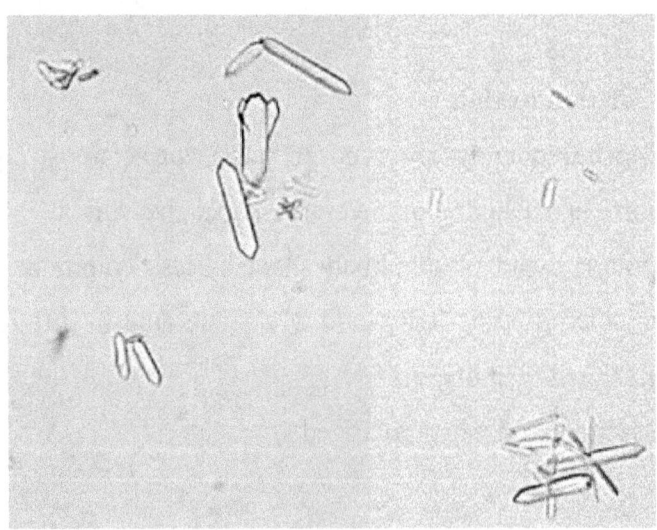

Normal crystals found in alkaline urine

1. Amorphous phosphates

❖ Non-crystalline form of phosphates resembles fine, colorless grains of sand.

❖ Sediment appears white; soluble in acid, does not dissolve at 60°C

❖ Very similar to amorphous urates; use pH to differentiate

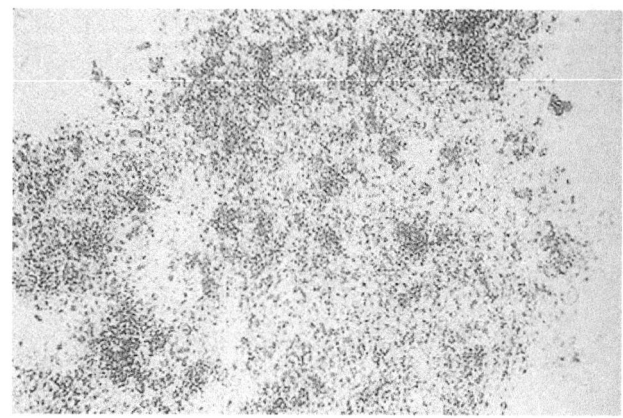

2. Triple phosphate

❖ Most common crystal seen in alkaline urine

❖ Colorless, 4 to 6-sided prisms resembling "coffin lids"; not all perfectly formed, and size varies

❖ Upon standing will begin to dissolve and appear feathery, resembling fern leaf

❖ Generally not clinically significant; associated with UTI (alkaline pH) and calculi formation

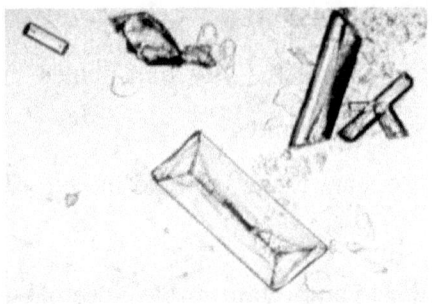

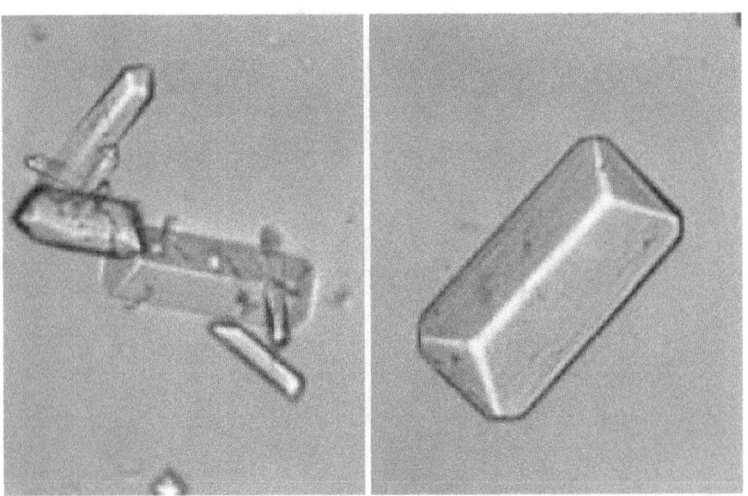

3. Calcium phosphate

❖ Distinctly different crystalline shapes: colorless thin wedge-like prisms arranged in rosettes or thin, long needles arranged in bundles or irregular, granular sheets/flat plates, latter form sometimes seen floating on top of urine specimen.

76

❖ Not clinically significant

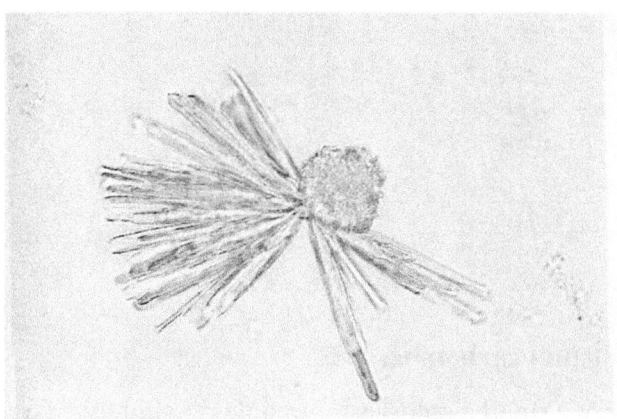

4. Ammonium biurate

❖ Yellow-brown spheres with striations on surface and irregular spicules (projections) giving a 'thorny apple' appearance

❖ Most often seen in urine improperly handled (prolonged storage) and clinically not significant

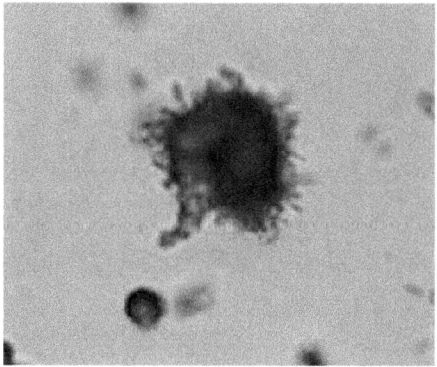

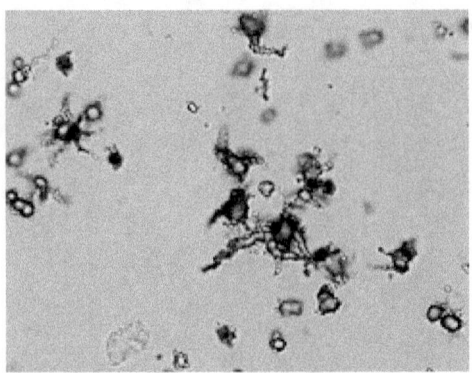

5. Calcium carbonate

❖ Very small colorless granules, slightly larger than amorphous material; often found in pairs giving them dumbbell shape

❖ Can be confused with bacteria

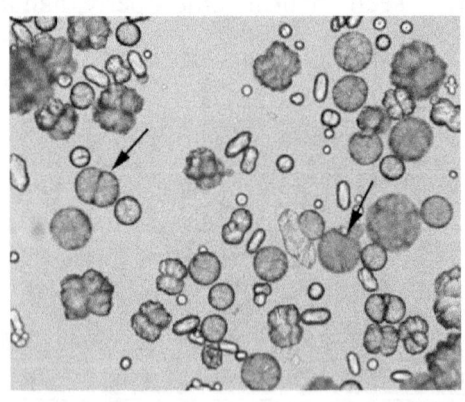

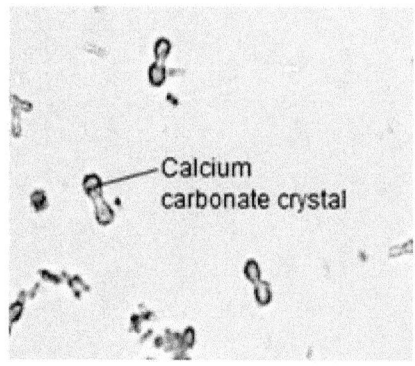

VI. Pathologic Crystals (acid, neutral pH)

1. Cystine Crystals

❖ Colorless hexagonal plates

❖ Do not polarize

❖ Can be confused with uric acid crystals

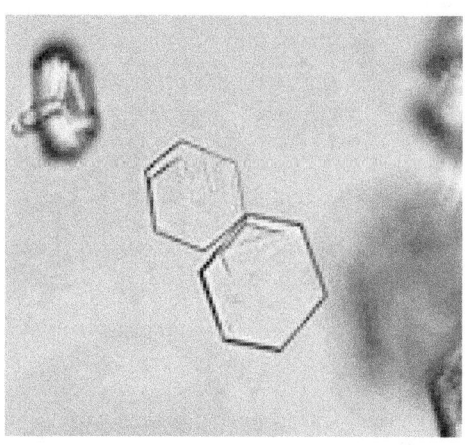

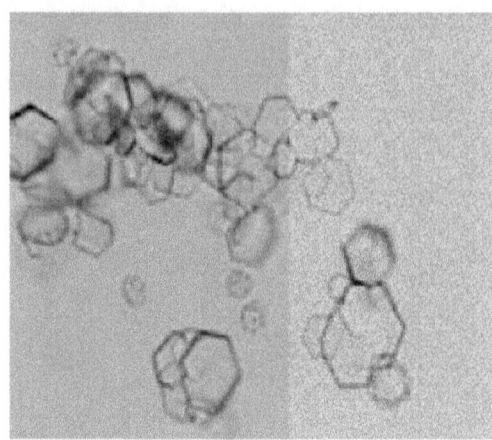

2. Cholesterol Crystals

❖ Clear, large, flat, rectangular plates with notched corners

❖ Multicolored when polarized

❖ Can be confused with radiographic dye crystals

❖ Also should see proteinuria and lipiduria

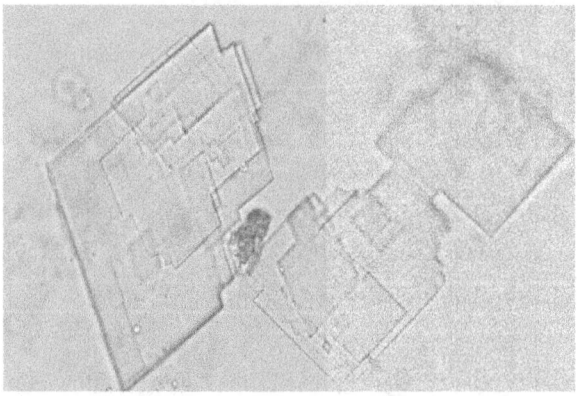

3. Leucine Crystals

❖ Yellow-brown spheres with concentric circles on surface (tree trunk)

❖ Can resemble free fat globules

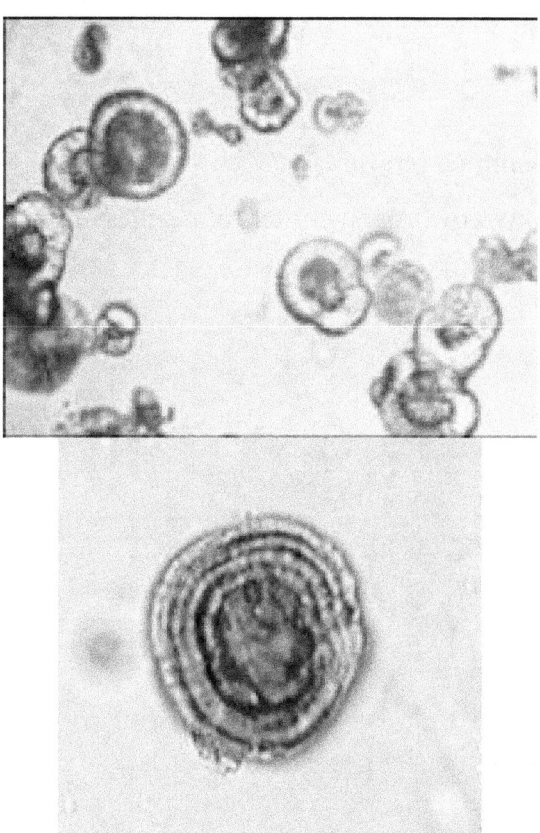

4. Tyrosine Crystals

❖ Colorless or yellow-brown fine delicate needles

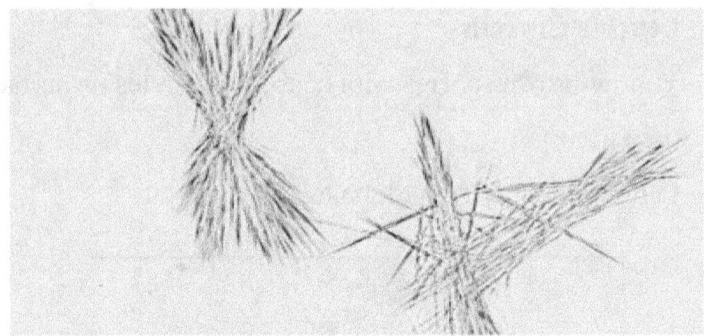

5. Bilirubin Crystals

❖ Yellow-brown small clusters of needles or granules

❖ Must confirm with positive Ictotest

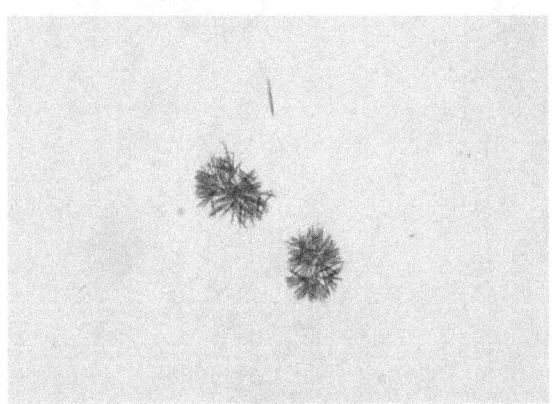

❖ Bilirubin: thicker needles, blunt ends

❖ Tyrosine: fine needles, pointy ends

VII. **Other microscopic elements**

1. **Bacteria**

❖ Most often see rod-shaped (bacilli) but can also see coccid forms; vary in size and shape; identified using **high power**

❖ Motility often differentiates bacteria from amorphous material

❖ Correlate with other results:

a. Reagent strip test: nitrites

b. pH often alkaline:

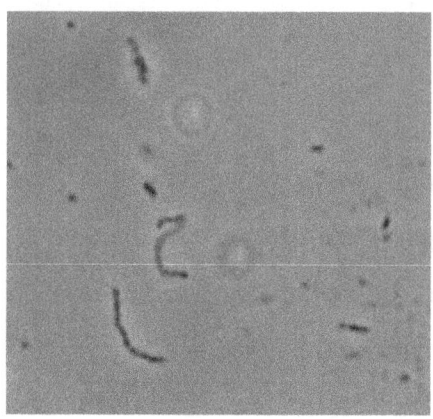

2. Yeast

❖ Ovoid, colorless cells; can resemble RBC (add 2% acetic acid to lyse RBC

❖ Yeast are more refractile than RBC, and often show budding forms and pseudohyphae (referred to as mycelial elements)

❖ Presence of yeast implies vaginal yeast infection with contamination of urine occurring during urine collection

❖ Yeast can be the primary cause of UTI (although rare)

❖ Most common is *Candida albicans* (show budding and pseudohyphae, referred to as mycelial elements)

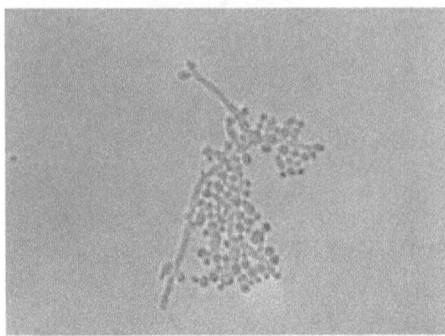

3. *Trichomonas vaginalis*

❖ Lemon/pear shaped protozoan flagellate

❖ Undulating membrane and flagella

❖ Characteristic flitting or jerky motion; once in urine, trichomonads begin to die, need fresh urine to identify

❖ Most common parasitic

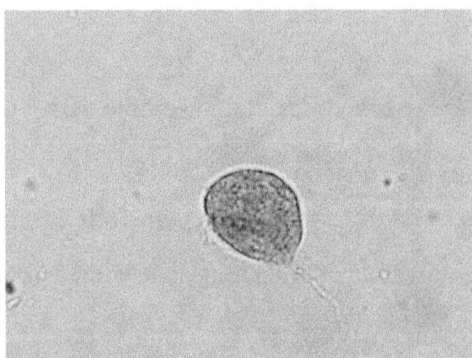

4. *Schistosoma haematobium* ova

❖ Introduced directly into urine from the bladder wall mucosa

❖ Parasitic infection, requires treatment

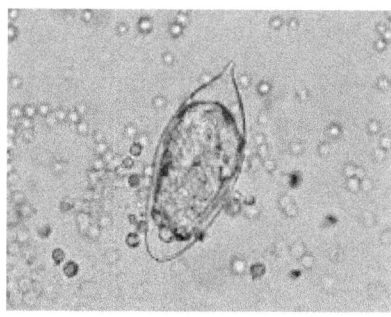

5. Spermatozoa

❖ May be seen in female and male urine

❖ Usually not clinically significant when found in urine

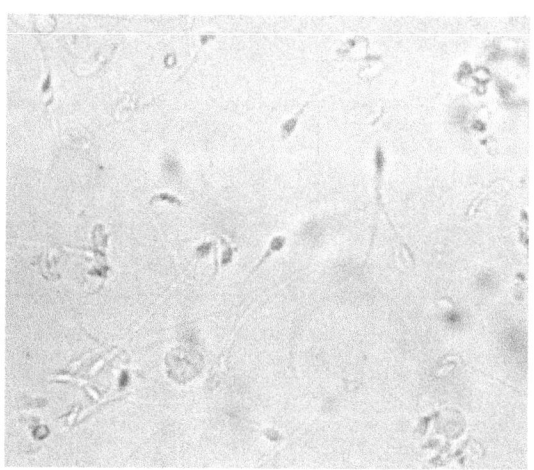

6. Mucus

❖ Wavy, delicate, ribbon-like strands with irregular or serrated ends.

❖ Low refractive index makes them difficult to see with Brightfield microscopy; identified on low power

❖ Can be mistaken for hyaline cast

- ❖ Produced in renal tubular epithelium, genitourinary tract and vaginal epithelium

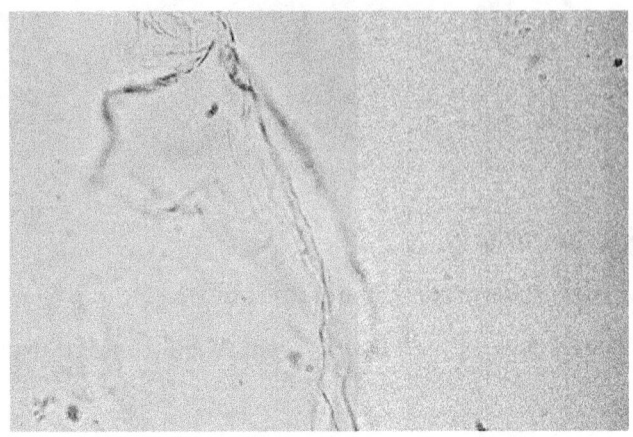

References

1. Assamenew, K., Mistir, W. & Belayhun, K., 2002. LECTURE NOTES For Medical Laboratory Technology Students Urinalysis. IndaBook.

2. CUMMER, C.L., 1932. A Manual of Clinical Laboratory Methods. J thessoc. Am. Med. Coll., 7(1), pp.63-64.

3. Fogazzi, G.B. & Garigali, G., 2003. The clinical art and science of urine microscopy. Curr Opin Nephrol Hypertens, 12, pp.625-32.

4. Free, H.M., ed., 1996. Modern Urine Chemistry (Manual). 8th ed. Bayer Corp.

5. Kaminskas, A. & Mažeikienė, A., 2012. BIOCHEMISTRY LABORATORY MANUAL. Vilnius University Faculty of Medicine.

6. Mundt, L. & Shanahan, K., 2010. raff's Textbook of Urinalysis and Body Fluids. 2nd ed. LWW.

7. Muruganathan, H., 2013. Section 17: Nephrology 127. Urinalysis in Clinical Practice 576 Sekhar Chakraborty. In MEDICINE UPDATE. JAYPEE BROTHERS MEDICAL PUBLISHERS PVT LTD.

8. Phillips, C.L., 1991. Basic laboratory procedure manual. pp.265-97.

9. Schumann, G.B. & Schweitzer, S.C., 1996. Examination of urine. In Clinical Chemistry, Theory, Analysis and Correlation. Third edition ed. St. Louis, Mosby-Year Book Inc.

10. Shihabi, Z.K., Konen, J.O. & O'Connor, M.L., 1991. Albuminuria vs urinary total protein for detecting chronic renal disorders. Clin Chem, 37, pp.621–24.

11. Strasinger, S.K. & Di Lorenzo, M.S., 2008. Urinalysis and Body Fluids. 5th ed. F A Davis.

12. University of Nebraska Medical Center, 2012. Routine Urinalysis- Microscopic Examination of Urine of Urine. Application and Interpretation.

13. Wanda, L., 2015. The Complete Urinalysis and Urine Tests. WWW.RN.ORG.

14. http://clinical-laboratory.blogspot.com.eg/2013/07/trichomonas-vaginalis-reviewing.html

15. http://cursoenarm.net/UPTODATE/contents/mobipreview.htm?13/26/13738

16. http://edusanjalbiochemist.blogspot.com.eg/2013/01/urinal
ysis-chemical-examination.html

17. http://equizshow.com/print/16739

18. http://pulpbits.net/8-white-blood-cells-in-urine-
pictures/white-blood-cells-casts-pictures/

19. http://studydroid.com/printerFriendlyViewPack.php?packId
=329821

20. http://uoitclinicalbiochemistry.weebly.com/urinalysis-
crystals.html

21. http://www.bd.com/vacutainer/labnotes/Volume14Number
2/

22. http://www.chromedia.org/chromedia?waxtrapp=sptlvLsH
onOvmOllEcCKD&subNav=wptlvLsHonOvmOllEcCKDn
C

23. http://www.eclinpath.com/urinalysis/crystals/calcium-
carbonate/

24. http://www.enjoypath.com/cp/Chem/Urine-
Morphology/Urine-morphology.htm

25. http://www.free-ed.net/free
ed/Courses/06%20MedHealth/MD%20Series/MD0852/Uri
nalysis.asp?iNum=0303

26. http://www.free-ed.net/free
ed/Courses/06%20MedHealth/MD%20Series/MD0852/Uri
nalysis.asp?iNum=0101

27. http://www.ivyroses.com/HumanBody/Urinary/Urinary_Sy
stem_Composition_Urine.php

28. http://www.med.illinois.edu/depts_programs/sciences/clini cal/internal_med/residency/edmod/mod1/casts.htm

29. http://www.med-health.net/Amorphous-Urates.html

30. http://www.medical-labs.net/red-blood-cells-casts-in-renal-hematuria-408/

31. http://www.microscopyu.com/articles/polarized/polarizedin tro.html

32. https://labtestsonline.org/understanding/analytes/urinalysis/ui-exams/start/1

33. https://memorize.com/first-aid-rapid-review-1-classic-presentations-jr--part-8/rujokehu

34. https://quizlet.com/12608416/urinalysis-final-flash-cards/

35. https://quizlet.com/87590982/urinecrystals-flash-cards/

36. https://www.studyblue.com/notes/note/n/kidney-1-b-/deck/5252306

ABOUT THE AUTHOR

Dr. Ayman Saber Mohamed was born in Giza, Egypt, in 1984. He received the B. Sc.degree in chemistry and zoology from faculty of science, Cairo University, Egypt, in 2011. He joined the Department of zoology, Faculty of science, Cairo University as a Demonstrator in 2013. In 2014, he got the M. Sc.degree and became teacher assistant of molecular and integrated physiology.

www.ingramcontent.com/pod-product-compliance
Lightning Source LLC
Chambersburg PA
CBHW061443180526
45170CB00004B/1530